You And Your Baby Can Sleep Through The Night

A Step by Step Manual for Exhausted Parents on How to Train Your Baby to Sleep Every Single Night in 7 days!

Harley Carr

entertainment purposes only. All effort has been executed to present accurate, up to date, reliable, complete information. No warranties of any kind are declared or implied. Readers acknowledge that the author is not engaging in the rendering of legal, financial, medical or professional advice. The content within this book has been derived from various sources. Please consult a licensed professional before attempting any techniques outlined in this book.

By reading this document, the reader agrees that under no circumstances is the author responsible for any losses, direct or indirect, that are incurred as a result of the use of the information contained within this document, including, but not limited to, errors, omissions, or inaccuracies.

Hello there Mommies,

Caring for your newborn brings great joy and excitement, but with it also comes sleep deprivation. It's a fact: Newborns simply can't sleep through the night, so neither can you.

The good news is that babies typically develop regular sleep patterns and can be put to sleep with help of a proper sleep-training As your baby's brain matures over these first few months, you'll probably see a sleep pattern start to emerge. Help your newborn establish a consistent sleep pattern by making routines for your baby's daily activities. In this way, you get back your sleep as well.

Track your baby's daily schedule for feeding, sleeping, crying and changing diapers. Once those patterns begin to form, you can help your baby settle into a daily routine and sleep pattern.

So, get you're your Your Baby Schedule Tracker " in PDF format by clicking the link below:

https://harleycarrparenting.com/you-and-your-baby-can-sleep-through-the-night/

+

QR Code

Print the document and start to record your Baby's daily Activities.

This Printable baby Schedule chart can help you identify patterns and figure out a routine that works for your baby and for the whole family.

Now, you can have your "Baby Schedule Tracker" in just one click away!

Let´s get started ...

Enjoy and Best Wishes to you Mommy!

Harley Carr

Table Of Contents

Introduction

You knew that bringing home your bundle of joy meant you wouldn't sleep well for a period of time, yet this time frame seems to never end. You are stressed. Your anxiety is worse than before. You are struggling to make your baby fall asleep and this is causing you more problems than you ever imagined. Your patience is thin, you can't make rational decisions, your work performance is low, and you are not getting along with a few of your family members. No matter what you have tried, you cannot get your baby to fall asleep. Nothing is working and you don't know what to do.

Fortunately, you have already taken the first step to help your baby fall asleep successfully every night, just by choosing this book. Here, we will discuss two of the best methods to help your baby fall asleep so you can get a good night's sleep too. Furthermore, you will learn the 10 habits that you need to avoid to ensure your baby sleeps promptly.

I am Harley Carr, and I am the mother of three children. Raising three kids is such a challenging role. I've been through a lot of difficulties during their first year of life, especially concerning their sleeping patterns and feeding schedules. I have been changing diapers for the last eight years! This is my life and I was able to manage them (of course with the help of my partner). I was lucky enough to survive those sleepless nights.

However, I also know that not everyone has a partner to help them. There are many great single parents out there who are in the same boat. This book will help you too. I remember many times where my best friend, a single parent, called me in the middle of the night ready to pull her hair out. She burst into tears so many times, as she wished so much that she didn't have to do it all alone. After taking on the 10 habits, which we are about to discuss, she successfully got her child to sleep every night.

To the mother who has twins or multiples, this book will not leave you out either. Your struggles are similar to the rest of us, yet special as you hold more than one baby. This gives extra challenges, ones that another friend of mine has discussed with me. They struggled with breastfeeding to the point that they felt they needed to give up. Because she and her partner worked different shifts, they each had to juggle two babies at the same time and it became nearly impossible, especially when they lacked patience due to sleep deprivation. She did continue to breastfeed, citing a twin pillow giving her the best support when breastfeeding.

This book is for the person or step-parent who doesn't have a child of their own but cares for another person's baby. Whether you are in a relationship with the baby's parent or you are a caregiver, you will learn ways to help the baby and everyone else in the situation receive a good night's sleep. Taking care of a child as a caregiver brings extra challenges as the baby is aware that their parents are not around. This

13

can add stress to the baby, which makes it more difficult for them to sleep. As long as everyone who will have the baby day and night is on the same page with sleep training, everyone can make this mission successful.

Here is an example of an alternative care situation in which both parties will need to be in sync with the sleep training procedure: Lisa is a newly single mom who recently left her husband after dealing with domestic abuse. Afraid that the baby's father will harm her son, she does what she can to ensure that she has their baby at all times. Her friend, Jasmine, decided to move out of the college dorms and into Lisa's new apartment to help her with the baby. Lisa, who is struggling with postpartum depression, is now facing a divorce and a loss of income. Falling into a deep depression, she is unable to sleep most nights because her baby doesn't sleep wel Jasmine does everything she can to care for t' baby during the night as well, but this is caus Jasmine to fall behind on schoolwork. Soon starts failing her exams and doesn't ge' assignments completed. Jasmine is afraid she will flunk out of school. She knows the baby isn't her responsibility, but she feels the need to help her best friend.

I am also writing to the parent who feels like they do it all, even when they have a partner. Your significant other might be out of town working, busy with long days at the office, or simply doesn't help out as much as you need them to. You might work at home and take care of your children. You do most (perhaps all) of the housework and are overstressed due to a lack of sleep.

Each one of us has a different story. But, no matter what your story is, I am talking to *you*. Together, we can help you overcome the struggle to get enough sleep. It doesn't matter who you are, what you believe, or how many people are in your family. Your family can consist of you and your baby, friends, other family members, a boyfriend, girlfriend, or fiance, *whatever*. You will receive the sleep training help needed to continue to grow your healthy family and environment.

In this book, I will share my insights and tips about how to cope and manage challenges and difficulties during your baby's first year and most importantly how to help them sleep soundly and consistently without compromising their health or physical and emotional development.

Once you've read this book, you will know what sleep training is and understand the steps you need to take so your baby sleeps through the night. You will learn when the time is right to start sleep training, what you need to expect, and how you should handle these expectations. We will discuss which sleep training method is the best for you, your baby, and your family. You will learn the secret sauce to sleep training and receive step-by-step guidelines to ensure your baby sleeps soundly every night. Furthermore, you will learn the 10 habits you need to avoid to make sleep training successful. You will not only get your baby to sleep well each night, but everyone else in the household will get quality shut-eye as well. Thus, you will think straight, your anxieties will dissipate, and you will make better decisions. Hold on, I haven't even mentioned the greatest part of this process yet— you will begin to really enjoy your role as a parent while maintaining great relationships with your partner, family, and friends.

My promise to you is that this book will fully equip you with the knowledge and skills you need to successfully sleep train your baby. You will set up the perfect feeding schedule to help your baby maintain a 24-hour routine. When your little one adapts to their new routine, they will sleep soundly throughout the night. This will have obvious positive effects for your baby, but also for you, and everyone else in the household.

At the moment, you feel like you are starting to lose your mind. You feel like your marbles have spilled and are rolling everywhere. You try to catch them, but all you do is kick them into more chaos as you chase them, just as you and your baby continue to struggle with the lack of sleep more and more despite your efforts. On top of this, you surely have other stressors in your life. You have no idea what to do and you feel like you have already done everything humanly possible. While some steps worked in the short-term, nothing is working long-term.

You might even be so desperate as to be looking at hiring a sleep consultant for 72-hours of in-house training. The biggest problem with this is that it is a stranger and they cost close to $7,500. You have a baby and other responsibilities and cannot afford to spend this type of money to help your baby sleep.

Good news—you don't need to look at a sleep consultant because *you* can take care of sleep training using the system in the contents of this book. Not only will this allow you to save money, but you will find the best solution for you personally in the following chapters. It will answer all of your questions and will give you the complete steps on how to train your baby to sleep every single night. Put simply: It will help you survive. You can escape those sleepless nights and avoid the harmful effects that sleep deprivation causes to babies and parents. These dangerous effects can:

- lead to obesity

- have a negative effect on the immune system

- disturb memory

- lower cognitive scores

- cause moodiness

- overstimulate your baby

- lead to inattention and hyperactivity

- increase separation anxiety

- delay the baby's growth

- make vaccinations less effective

- lead to long-term social and emotional problems

- possibly be linked to autism

- reduce parents' patience

- reduce parental focus

- lead to fatal consequences when a parent is too sleep-deprived

Don't wait for another night. Read on for the absolute best sleep training advice, so everyone in your household can finally get a much-deserved good night's sleep!

Chapter 1: What Is Sleep Training and What Are the Harmful Effects of Sleep Deprivation?

Sleep Training

Sleep training is a process that has become more common over the last several years. It is when you help your baby learn how to soothe themselves to sleep and stay asleep for the rest of the night.

It is important to note that babies will learn sleep training at different intervals. Some babies will fall asleep easily while other babies will struggle to soothe themselves into a deep sleep. There is also the possibility of your baby falling asleep quickly but still waking up in the middle of the night and having a hard time getting themselves back to sleep. No matter how your child reacts to sleep training, they will all need help to learn the process.

When can I start sleep training?

There is a lot of debate on what is the best age to start sleep training your baby. Some people say that you should begin as soon as they come home from the hospital. However, most experts will tell you to wait until your baby is four months old. You want your little one to develop regular nightly feedings and a sleep-wake schedule, or at least as much as possible before you begin training. Once you start noticing that your baby is on a bit of a cycle, you can start sleep training. Remember, each baby is an individual and this means they will all vary in sleep characteristics too. For instance, you and your friend start sleep training at the same time. You notice your friend's baby is quickly learning to soothe themselves to sleep, but your baby is still struggling. In this case, your baby might not be ready for sleep training. They might also need less sleep and are not as tired when you start to get them ready for bed.

You should always communicate with your baby's doctor when you are thinking about starting sleep training. Let the doctor know your plan as this is something you can update them with throughout the process. This is helpful for all parents, but especially single parents as it gives you another person to support you during this time. Emotional and psychological support can help ease any problems that arise and make you more confident in the sleep training process.

How to prepare for sleep training

To help you prepare for sleep training, you should follow these tips:

- **Choose a consistent bedtime.** One of the first steps in getting your baby ready for sleep training is to set a bedtime. Experts state that the best time for your baby is between 7:00 and 8:00. You might already have a time that you follow, but not as closely as you should. If you decide to lay your baby down for bed at 7:30 p.m. you need to stick to this time as much as possible. Keep in mind, life is unpredictable, and you will most likely have days that you can't lay your baby down directly at this time. For example, you are driving home from a family member's house after an emergency situation. In this case, your baby might fall asleep on their own as you drive, which can cause problems as you wake them up to bring them inside for bed. The key to a slight change in their routine is to remain calm and realize it happens. As long as you are consistent with their bedtime in the following nights, your baby will not be affected by one late bedtime.

- **Establish a bedtime routine.** You should start a bedtime routine before you begin sleep training. Most experts say you can start a routine at four weeks old, but don't worry if you haven't started a routine and your child is older—simply create the routine and begin. It is never too late! Your routine can be anything from giving your little one a nice warm bath to reading a short book. You might sing a song or speak to them about your day in a soothing voice. No matter what you decide, you want to make sure it is calming and relaxes your baby.

- **Ensure your baby does not have a medical condition that may affect their sleep.** This is one reason it is important to talk to your baby's doctor before you start sleep training. The pediatrician can perform an exam to make sure your baby doesn't suffer from any type of medical condition that can keep them from getting a good night's sleep. If you find out that they do, follow the doctor's orders to give your baby the best success rate for sleep training.

- **Establish a daytime schedule that you can follow.** A daytime routine is just as important as a bedtime routine. Ensure that you lay your baby down for a nap at the set times, follow a feeding schedule, and keep them busy throughout the day so they are more tired when it is time for bed. The more secure your baby feels the more success you and your baby will have with sleep training.

What are my sleep training options?

There are many sleep training options, but we will focus on two of the main methods:

1. **Cry it out method.** The cry it out method is one of the most debatable approaches because some people don't understand this method. Many people feel it leaves your baby to cry in their crib

until they fall asleep. This is not true. While your baby will most likely start crying when you start sleep training, you want to have a set time for the cry it out method. For instance, you might allow your baby to cry for a couple of minutes before you go back in there and comfort them, without picking them up. Once they calm down, you will leave the room again and wait to see if they fall asleep. If they are still crying after a couple of minutes, you go back into the room to comfort them as they continue to lay in their crib. For example, you might rub their back and hum softly.

2. **No tears method.** In this method, you will comfort your child immediately when they start crying. This is a gradual approach that will give you the same results as the cry it out method.

Harmful Effects of Sleep Deprivation

You know how sleep deprivation can affect you. Take a minute to think about how it can affect your baby. You might think that your little one is getting enough sleep. After all, they seem to sleep all the time, especially when they are only a few months old. However, about 30% to 40% of children are not getting the sleep they need (15 Ways Lack of Sleep Is Harmful To The Baby, 2016).

There are many reasons for sleep deprivation in babies and it can be hard to know if they are overtired because they can't directly tell you. But don't worry, they will let you know in other ways. Here are some symptoms of sleep deprivation your baby might exhibit:

- You have trouble feeling your baby.

- They rub their eyes often.

- Their eyelids flutter a lot.

- They yawn often.

- They seem easily irritable.

- They are not interested in their surroundings or other people.

- You notice your baby is scared of bedtime. This is a symptom most commonly seen in older babies.

- They don't sleep often during the day or you notice a decrease in the amount of time they sleep that does not correspond to their age.

- You notice your baby pauses breathing while they are sleeping.

You need to be aware that you will see one of two of these signs now and then. For example, if your baby had a difficult night falling asleep or didn't sleep well this causes them to yawn, rub their eyes, and they won't want to eat like they normally do. Because these symptoms are not every day, there is no need to worry. Your child will get a better night's sleep the next night. If you start to notice these symptoms every day for a couple of weeks, then you will want to visit your baby's pediatrician.

Now that you understand the symptoms of sleep deprivation in babies, now we'll explore how else it can affect your baby.

Can cause obesity

Babies who don't get the necessary sleep are more likely to become overweight by three years old. Sleeping affects many parts of the body and mind, including your baby's metabolism. It becomes slower with a lack of sleep, which makes your baby gradually increase weight. The extra weight gain happens because of an imbalance of energy which affects several hormones, such as leptin, insulin, growth, and ghrelin.

Johns Hopkins University completed a study that showed that an extra hour of sleep a baby receives during night decreases their chance of obesity by 9%, whereas a baby who sleeps less than their needed time increase their chances of obesity by 92% (15 Ways Lack of Sleep Is Harmful To The Baby, 2016).

Negatively affects their immune system

Children who do not receive the sleep they need are more likely to become ill because their immune system suffers. It is easier for a baby to catch the flu or cold when they do not get the sleep they need. The UCLA Cousins Center conducted a study that showed even a small amount of sleep loss can negatively affect the immune system. It causes tissue damage and triggers inflammation (Elsevier, 2008).

One of the best ways to fight off bacteria growing in a baby's body happens while your baby is sleeping. Disease fighting proteins are released from the immune system, but they can only be released when sleeping. Therefore, the longer your baby is awake, the fewer proteins their immune system will produce. With a lack of proteins, it is also harder for your baby to fight off any illness that enters their system, which means they are sick for a longer duration.

This can happen whether your baby loses an hour of sleep a week or an hour every night. But, the longer your baby goes without the necessary amount of sleep, the more serious this effect becomes. Therefore, if your baby is showing signs of sleepiness, especially on a regular basis, you need to take the time to increase their amount of sleep every night.

Disturbs memory

You know how much you struggle mentally when you don't get a good night's sleep. Your baby will also struggle in this way when they don't get the sleep they need. A lack of sleep impairs functioning within the brain, causing difficulty in learning and impairs memory. Your baby is learning every day. They might not remember what they see as a baby when they grow older, but they are still learning and taking in their scenery, nonetheless. They are learning who to trust and about their surroundings.

When your baby suffers from a lack of sleep, they cannot comprehend their environment strongly. They will struggle to store memories as they do not get enough Random Eye Movement (REM) sleep, which consists of 50 to 80% of their sleep (15 Ways Lack of Sleep Is Harmful To The Baby, 2016). Professors at the University of Arizona conducted a study that focused on memory and sleep of babies at 15 months old. For 15 minutes, the babies listened to a fake language recording. Four hours later, the professors tested all babies and found that the ones who napped prior to testing remembered the recording better. Furthermore, they became more flexible in learning. The babies who did not nap before testing did not remember the recording at all.

Lowers cognitive scores

With the disturbance of memory, it is not surprising that a lack of sleep also lowers your cognitive scores. A child's brain is constantly developing, and this means less sleep can permanently affect your baby's mind. Researchers at the University of Colorado concluded through a study that the brain forms new cell connections when a child is sleeping. In fact, the left and right brain forms close to 20% of its connections during sleep (15 Ways Lack of Sleep Is Harmful To The Baby, 2016).

One of the best ways to ensure that your baby will get enough sleep is to give them an early bedtime. Think of the amount of time it takes your child to fall asleep and when they should fall asleep to make certain they get the amount of time they need. For example, a five-month-old baby should sleep 12 to 15 hours in a 24-hour period. If your baby naps two hours a day, this means they need at least 10 hours of sleep at night. You put your baby to bed at 7:30 p.m., but they never fall asleep until about 8:30 p.m. You need to get your baby up at 5:30 a.m. to get them ready for daycare so you can go to work. This means, at most, your baby gets eight or nine hours of sleep, falling below the recommended 10. Because your baby takes about an hour to fall asleep, you want to put them to bed at 6:30 p.m. They will fall asleep by 7:30 p.m. and get at least 12 hours of sleep every day.

Makes your baby moody

There is something that you can never truly control with your baby—their moodiness. It is something that everyone struggles with, but most adults can control their moods. This is something that your baby cannot control because they simply do not have the ability yet. Therefore, you need to do everything you can to help your baby's moodiness and, thankfully, one of the biggest steps you can take is sleep training.

When your baby does not get the sleep they need, they get fussy and frustrated quickly. While most babies will cry easily, they tend to bounce back quickly. If you notice your baby cries for several minutes or you struggle to get them to calm down, your baby might be sleep-deprived.

Overstimulation

Like you, when your baby does not get enough sleep, they become overtired. When this happens, they become overstimulated and this makes it harder for them to fall asleep. Overstimulation causes more stress on your baby, which causes them to become moody and more prone to fits. Your baby can't bring themselves out of this situation, they need help and the best way to do this is by making sure they get the sleep they need for their age.

Hyperactivity and inattention

You know you lack focus when you do not get enough sleep and your baby is the same way. However, the difference between you and your baby is you lack energy and they gain energy. Sleep-deprived babies tend to become hyperactive. It is important to be cautious of your baby's sleep schedule before you or a doctor starts to wonder if your hyperactive baby is developing ADHD or ADD. Hyperactivity because a baby is overtired and symptoms of ADHD are often confused. The best factor to look at when you are trying to distinguish between the two is that children are usually older when doctors diagnose them with ADHD. You should also keep an eye out for other symptoms of tiredness such as rubbing their eyes and moodiness.

Increases separation anxiety

Once your baby understands object permanence, they will develop separation anxiety. Separation anxiety is when they throw a fit, cry, or struggle when they realize you are no longer in their sight. Separation anxiety usually starts around nine to 10 months of age but can develop as early as six months old. Your baby can develop separation anxiety after sleep training, but it is more common for babies who are sleep deprived. Studies prove that babies who get the sleep they need have an easier time self-soothing when they are alone (15 Ways Lack of Sleep Is Harmful To The Baby, 2016).

Slow growth

Even though you do not always see it, your baby is constantly growing mentally, emotionally, and physically. Every day is a learning experience for them, and these situations help them grow in various ways. Babies who do not get the amount of sleep they need will develop at a slower rate than babies who do get the sleep they need. All types of growth are disturbed from their height to their developmental milestones. When a baby sleeps, about 8% of the somatotropin growth hormone is released. When a baby does not get the amount of sleep they need, this percentage drops.

Vaccinations are less effective

According to a study by the University of Pittsburgh School of Medicine, vaccines are not as effective for sleep-deprived babies. This study noted that the vaccine produced 12% fewer antibodies in babies who were sleep-deprived (15 Ways Lack of Sleep Is Harmful To The Baby, 2016).

Long-term emotional and social problems

When a child is sleep-deprived, they will avoid social activities because they feel it requires too much effort to interact with other people. They will also struggle with expressing themselves, whether it is verbally or nonverbally. Lack of sleep creates more negative emotions and makes children less likely to remember positive experiences. Your baby might feel more stressed and then have trouble learning new skills, making them fall behind in comparison with their peers. If your baby doesn't get the sleep they need for a long period of time, anxiety and depression can develop.

Might be linked to autism

Over the last several years, researchers have looked into what causes autism as it is on the rise in children. While scientists continue to find out the causes of autism, as many are relatively unknown, it is noted in their studies that sleep-deprived children have a higher risk of developing autism. A study conducted by psychologist Terry Katz and neurologist Beth Malow concluded that children who had autism, but no other health problems, could manage some of their symptoms when they received more sleep. Not only did their repetitive behavior decrease, but so did their anxiety.

Lack of patience for parents

There will always be moments where you feel frustrated as a parent. However, parents tend to have more frustrating moments when their baby is sleep-deprived. Because your child is exhibiting moodiness, struggling to focus, hyperactive, and overstimulated you become easily frustrated after they show these types of behaviors regularly or for a long period of time. Your patience wears thin over time as this is a human trait. Ensuring that your baby gets the sleep they need can help decrease the frustrating behaviors and give yourself more patience.

Parents lack focus

When your baby does not get the sleep they need it makes you sleep deprived as well. This will affect your focus and ability to monitor the many needs of your baby. For example, you might not realize that the formula is too hot or that the temperature of your baby's room is too cold. It is easy to lose focus on specific tasks and duties when you are tired.

Fatal consequences of parental sleepiness

It seems not a day goes by where you do not hear about a road accident. However, what you do not hear is about these accidents is that 1,000 fatal road accidents happen annually due to a lack of sleep. Because you lose patience quickly, you are tired, emotionally and mentally drained, and you lose focus you are more likely to end up in an accident.

Drowsy driving is just as bad as drunk driving. If you are feeling tired, take time to take a 10 to 15-minute nap before you get on the road. If you are driving and feel that it is getting hard to keep your eyes open, pull over in a parking lot or safely on the side of the road and rest your eyes. Call a friend or family member if you need someone else to drive you home safely.

Chapter 2: Family Structure (Teamwork Works!)

Your family can consist of many people, friends, blood relatives, neighbors and maybe even coworkers. However, no matter who your family consists of, it is important to realize the importance of them and the teamwork they can offer.

No matter what your role is in the family, you need to remember the word "teamwork" because it really does work. To ensure your baby gets the most out of sleep training, every member needs to work together. Even if you have a babysitter for the night, you need to make sure they understand your baby's routine. Walkthrough the routine with them and leave a note that shows the babysitter the steps of the routine. Some parents like to place pictures of their child's bedtime routine on the child's wall. When the child is older, they can look at the picture and understand what is next in the routine.

For this chapter, we will focus on three different structures within your family: dad, grandparents, and a partner. Each person will play a significant role in your baby's life and help ensure that sleep training works for you, your baby, and your family.

Role of Dads

American society often places the role of the dad in the family on the sidelines. We still live in a world where the mother is thought of as the nurturer and the main parent for the children. Fortunately, this view is starting to change dads. In fact, there are a number of dads who want to do everything they can to help their baby adjust during the sleep training period.

If you have a family with a dad, they must become just as important in the sleep training process as you. Forget about what society has told you when it comes to dads in the parenting relationship. They can do nearly everything you can do. They can also be your sense of support during the difficult moments, such as the nights where your baby is teething and sleeping their normal number of hours is becoming more and more difficult. But, with the support of your baby's dad, you can make it through these nights.

The dad does not need to live in the same house as the mom to take part in sleep training. If there are two different homes, communicate with each other and come to an agreement on what is the best sleep training routine for your baby. Be respectful of each other and follow through with the plan. Remember, slacking in one home because one of you does not agree with every step of sleep training will harm the child more than anyone else. It is always best to keep the baby in a routine.

Here are a few tips to include in the sleep training when it comes to the dad's role:

- **The baby's dad can help put them back to sleep at any age.** Some people believe that when breastfeeding, the mom always needs to get up and put the baby back to sleep, but this is not necessarily true. A mother can always prepare the milk for the nighttime and the dad can bottle feed. Another way dads can help is to get up during the feeding and then burp the child when the baby is done with feeding. This will allow the mother to go to bed a get a bit more sleep. Furthermore, when your baby is starting to wean from breastfeeding, they will continue to wake up at certain times during the night out of habit. Dads can easily take a turn to soothe their baby back to sleep.

- **Dads are great at being a shoulder to cry on.** Sleep training, even when you do your best to remain calm, is hard. You will feel stressed at times and you might even have moments where you think, "I can't do this anymore." These are some of the best moments to talk to the baby's father. They will understand where you are coming from and offer you support. There is nothing wrong with venting about the process as this can help you remain consistent and keep everyone focused on the goal.

- **Include dads into the bedtime routine.** You can always take turns when it comes to the bedtime routine. For example, you might give the baby a bath and the dad might read to them. Then, you both put your baby to bed by tucking them in and telling them goodnight. You can both take part in the bedtime routine every step of the way as well. Don't think that the steps need to be split or one should do most of the steps and then both of the parents tuck the baby in.

- **Take time to feed the baby with a bottle.** Not all babies are breastfed and if your baby takes the bottle, then the dad can take charge of some of the nightly feedings. You might decide between you to take turns or focus on what is best when it comes to your work schedules.

Role of Grandparents

Grandparents are great to lean on when it comes to sleep training. While they might have their own ideas on how to sleep train a baby, grandparents are great people to look to when you need some emotional or psychological support. They have been in your shoes and understand how stressful it is to sleep train a child. Even if they didn't sleep train, they understand the difficulties in getting a baby to sleep through the night and will understand when you need a shoulder to cry on.

It is important to remember when considering grandparents as support is that you might need to speak up and ask if they will help you. Some grandparents will jump at the chance to help and will constantly ask you if you need anything, while other grandparents will give you space and wait for you to come to them. By now, you understand the grandparents better than anyone else. But no matter what your relationship is like with them, you always need to take time to explain the process to them.

Understand that grandparents grew up in a different time and if they criticize your methods, they are not trying to hurt you. They might feel their advice will help you. Listen to what they have to say and do your best to explain your process. Try to get them to understand the importance of consistency and be patient. Your baby's grandparents have the best interest at heart for your baby and they will do what they need to.

No matter what your relationship is with the grandparents, you need to focus on the special relationship between your baby and their grandparents. Here are a few factors about their special relationship:

- **Love is unconditional.** There is nothing that your child could do that will make the grandparents stop loving them. This is the same love that you feel for your child.

- **It is usually more carefree.** Grandparents have already raised their children and now they want to focus on the fun part and be a grandparent. This can help you greatly, especially if they will take time to rock your baby before bed or get up in the middle of the night to soothe your baby back to sleep. Most grandparents have more patience for their grandchildren than you have for your child. This isn't bad, it is typical when it comes to this relationship dynamic.

- **They might have more time.** Grandparents might be retired and do not have the same day-to-day tasks and responsibilities that you do. This allows them to stay with the baby and make sure that they are following their schedule while you are working or running errands.

Share Sleep Training With a Partner

The first step to sleep training with your partner is to get on the same page. Whether you are roommates, married, dating, or co-parenting, you and your partner need to have strong communication skills in order to effectively sleep train. Sit down and talk about the sleep training schedule, the nighttime routine, and the best time to lay your baby down to sleep. You need to have a bedtime that works for both of you, especially when tag-teaming the sleep training process. You both need to agree on which sleep training method you'll be applying to. If your partner is not sure they can listen to your baby cry for some time, for example, you'll probably opt for the no tears method.

Decide if you will split the sleep training responsibilities evenly with your partner or if you will hold most of the responsibilities. Every situation is different, and you need to find what works best for you and your family.

Go through the process together (without your baby) before you start sleep training to make sure that you both understand the process completely. Walk and talk it out from start to finish. For instance, if the bedtime routine starts with a warm bath, walk into the bathroom and discuss the length of the bath. Then move on to the next step. Will you have pajamas ready for your baby to put on in the bathroom or will you bring them into their bedroom? Continue this practice run through all the steps in your sleep training process.

Finally, choose a convenient date to start the sleep training process. You should start your training strong, so it is imperative that the first week works for both of your schedules.

Chapter 3: Multiple Births (Twins)

Every parent of twins or multiples will tell you that taking care of more than one baby is a monumentally bigger challenge. There is a lot of truth to this, especially if you are a single-parent household. While two parents can switch time with the twins and do their best to take care of feeding, diaper changes, and attention together, it is harder when you are the only parent taking care of two babies. There are also other factors involved if you are a parent to triplets or more babies. You can get a sense of how difficult trying to manage more than one baby can be when you only have one child to care for.

Taking Care of Two Babies

Personally, I can only imagine what it is like to take care of two babies. My experience comes from caring for my own children and watching my friend care for her twins. Of course, I have also checked out a couple of reality shows on raising multiples, but this doesn't compare to a parent or parents who take care of their twins every day.

One of the first questions that might come to your mind when caring for twins is, "How can I make this easier?" Chances are, you have already tried everything you can think of and some steps might have helped, but there are still several struggles you need to face. You are stressed and looking for help to alleviate your challenges.

First, it is important to remember that you are not alone in this category. Every new parent, even when they have a partner, can use more support. In fact, there is never enough support for parents. With this in mind, if you do have a partner, you need to remember that they don't have enough support to give you. Even if they help you with your babies with every feeding, your partner might also feel like they still haven't given enough help. Therefore, blaming each other will not help the situation. You need to support each other and recognize how much you are both doing as much and as often as you can.

If you start to feel your stress building, plan ahead so you can take a break or get some extra help for a couple of days. This might mean you contact your parents, in-laws, siblings, friends, or ask your insurance company if they will pay for a home nurse or night nurse to come and visit.

Breastfeeding may become another struggle when it comes to parenting multiples. You need to find a method that works for you. Some parents will get a twin nursing pillow to help them feed their twins at the same time. Of course, this method is not always possible. Sometimes, you need to feed your babies at different times, and this can cause problems when it comes to napping and bedtime. Take a few deep breaths and remember, these struggles are temporary.

Another tip when it comes to taking care of multiples is to take as much maternity leave as possible. You will need this to help get into your groove and take care of your babies. Some parents combine their vacation with maternity leave. Other parents will make sure that if their baby is sick that their Human Resources department knows this as then they might get a few extra days by using their sick time instead of maternity or vacation.

Finally, get a good foundation of support—not just from your friends and family. Find other parents with multiples in your area or online who you can talk to. They understand what you are going through and will have ideas that you can try with your family. Psychologically, when we know that other people understand our situation, we can handle every day a little easier because we know that we are not alone. Let me repeat, so you always remember this—you are not alone.

How to Sleep Train Twins

Most of the resources you receive about sleep training focus on caring for one baby, but sleep training multiples is just as important.

One of the first steps you need to accomplish is whether your twins will sleep together or apart. You might wonder if it is common for your babies to disturb each other when they are sleeping or if they will sleep better when they are co-sleeping, which is sleeping in the same bed. A few studies show that a little over half of the parents allow their babies to co-sleep, at least for the first couple of months. Many other parents will place the cribs next to each other so their twins can still comfort each other but have their own space.

The research of co-bedding twins comes up with a lot of debate, even from the experts. Some people believe it is healthy for your multiples, especially in the first few months. Twins are used to being next to each other, as they were in the womb. Other experts state that because there are no real benefits shown with co-sleeping and that it is best to ensure your twins each have their own crib. The bottom line is you need to do what you feel is right for you, your twins, and your family. If you do decide to co-bed, there are several ways that you can do this. Some people like to lay their babies side by side while other people will lay them head to head or feet to feet. No matter what you decide, the best step to take is to make sure they have enough room for themselves. They will be aware of their twins and won't harm or hit their sibling.

To help ease your worries about sleep training twins, here are some tips to follow:

- You don't need to place any type of barrier between your babies when they are co-sleeping. Barriers can hurt babies more than help them.

- The risk of SIDS for twins declines if they room-share or sleep in the same room with you for the first six months.

- Always lay babies on their backs when they are going to sleep. This will reduce the risk of SIDS.

Sleep patterns in twins are a bit different because they follow their gestational pattern over age, especially if they are born prematurely. Other than this, the way they sleep and how you will sleep train twins is similar to a single baby. For instance, you will develop a plan and find out what method will work best for you and your family. The biggest difference is that you have two (or more) babies instead of one. Most parents of multiples state that one of the best steps you can follow when you are sleep training is to do your best to feed and put your babies down to sleep at the same time. This might not be possible, especially if you are a single parent and struggle with feeding your twins at the same time. Do your best and your babies will fall into a routine, especially if you remain consistent.

Routines are just as important as multiples as they are with twins. Studies show that parents with multiples are more likely to follow a routine and receive help from other people. However, the amount of sleep deprivation that mothers have is the same whether they have one baby or more than one.

What to Expect and When

In reality, it is hard to know exactly what to expect and when each baby is different. They tend to follow their own schedule when it comes to growth and this can affect sleep training. The main goal for most parents with twins is to get your babies on the same schedule, especially when it comes to sleeping. Fortunately, sleep training will help.

Twins who are born prematurely will need more sleep during the first few weeks. It is also important to note that if your twins are born early, you might need to push back sleep training for a few weeks or so. For example, most parents will start sleep training once they receive approval from their child's pediatrician, which is usually between four to six months. But, if your twins were born a couple of months early, they won't be ready at the average time. You need to focus on their gestational age over actual age, so you might not start sleep training until between six to eight months.

To get your babies established in a routine, here are a few tips for you to follow:

- **Double-duty feedings.** It isn't easy, but you want to do what you can to make sure your babies eat at the same time as this will give them a stronger chance of falling asleep around the same time.

- **Have your babies nap at the same time.** Whether you decide to co-bed your twins or give them their own crib, you want to lay them down at the same time. One might be a bit drowsier than the other, but the other twin will quickly catch up.

- **Establish a good bedtime routine.** You might start with a bath as this will get your babies to understand that the sound of their bath means it is soon bedtime. After bath time, you want to ensure that you are playing soothing music or read them a story quietly. Doing something that is relaxing will help your babies fall asleep and stay asleep.

- **If one baby wakes up to eat, wake the other baby.** Of course, it will be hard to wake up your peacefully sleeping baby but doing so will keep your babies on the same schedule. Plus, once you get the twin who is up and eating to sleep, the other twin will wake up and they will continue to take turns throughout the night. This will mean, whether you are a single parent or have the help of a partner, you will get little to no sleep. Furthermore, the twins can keep waking each other up, which means you will have two tired and crabby babies the next day.

- **Establish small goals.** Chances are you have a lot of goals when it comes to keeping your twins on the same schedule. While this is great, the trick is to make sure that you establish small goals. Remember, your babies are usually a bit behind a single baby, especially if they are born prematurely. Keeping your goals small will help your babies thrive and keep you from becoming stressed because you are not where you want to be. Always get excited over the smallest achievements, such as feeding twice a night instead of three times.

- **If one twin sleeps through the night, it is okay to separate.** You will want to notice how your twins adjust if you decide to separate them into different rooms, but many parents do this as one twin might start sleeping through the night before the other twin. When this happens, it is a good idea to look at moving your little sleeper into a different room, even if it is the living room, because this will allow them to continue sleeping through the night. You can always move them back into their bedroom when the other twin is sleeping just as well.

The best routine and feeding schedule for twins

Even the most energetic mom can become overwhelmed by constantly waking up to feed her twins at different times. Plus, daily life with babies, even one, is chaotic and this only increases when you have twins. Placing your babies on a schedule will help them as they will sleep, eat, and play together. It will also help your emotional, mental, and physical health, which is extremely important. If you don't take care of yourself, it is harder to take care of your little ones.

While you want to keep your twins on the same schedule, you also need to be flexible. Don't keep your nodding your baby up if they are starting to fall asleep while the other twin continues to coo and interact with you. If one becomes hungry, don't force them to wait to eat until the other becomes hungry. Go ahead and give your little one a snack. Remaining flexible will allow you to attend to the needs of your babies individually, which is extremely important. You might have one twin that is more sensitive and needs more sleep and cuddles and one twin who shows more independence and doesn't need to sleep as much.

Through your flexibility and doing what you can to follow a schedule you set, your babies will start to follow the schedule over time. It might take several months and a lot longer than one baby, but this is how it works with twins. Following the cues of your twins will help them thrive.

Bath time

Splashing in the bath is double the fun when you have multiples. While some parents feel they can only bathe one baby at a time, as bathing just one baby is an intimidating task, to begin with, it is still best to bathe your twins together when they reach a certain age. Because newborns are more fragile, it is best to bathe them separately. Once you feel your babies are ready to take a bath at the same time, here are some tips to help you and your babies adjust:

- **Forget the bath seats.** Bath seats can tip when your baby is in the tub. They tend to give parents a false sense of security. While it might feel nice to have the extra help from the seats, nothing is better than your constant supervision. Plus, they make the bath less fun as they restrict your babies.

- **Start bathing them together when they can sit up without assistance.** Your babies will tell you when they are ready to take a bath together and this is when they can sit up without your assistance. When you start bathing them, you will want to have a slip-proof mat, always be within grabbing reach, and only have about two to three inches of water.

- **Your twins might go through phases where you need to split them.** Some babies enjoy getting their hair washed while other babies dislike this part. If one of your babies cries because they are getting their hair washed and this upsets the other twin, you might want to look at splitting them up for bath time. Continuing this process while they are together can cause them to dread bath time, which should always be a fun, relaxing activity.

- **Prepare for post-bath.** Chances are you will only take one twin out at a time, so you want to ensure you are prepared with a towel, pajamas, and a bouncy seat ready for the first twin to come up. Don't place the babies too far away from you. Remember, you always want to be in close contact so you can grab them in case they fall.

Problem-Solving (How to Deal with Your Crying Twin)

The way babies communicate is with their cries. As a parent, you start to learn what your baby's cries mean. You will learn they have a cry when they are hungry, a different cry when they are overtired, when they are scared, etc. While it is never fun to hear your baby cry, especially when they are having trouble calming down, it is normal. However, this doesn't mean it isn't stressful, especially for new parents and parents with more than one baby.

One factor you should be aware of is that there are no studies to prove multiples cry more than a single baby. It might seem this way at times, especially if your twins take turns crying, but it doesn't mean that you need to hear them cry more. What determines how often your baby cries depends on their personality. Sensitive babies will cry more because they are more sensitive to sound, touch, light, etc. When your baby is more laid back, they will cry less. Each baby will have their own special personality, and this means one twin might cry more than the other.

So what can you do when your baby is crying and you can't seem to calm them down? First, you want to remain as calm as possible. While this is not easy, it is the first step to calming a baby. Both of your babies can sense how you feel and if you feel stressed, they will begin to feel uneasy and both can become inconsolable, which will not help the situation. Here are a few more tips to help you soothe your crying babies:

- **Set your babies together.** If you don't co-bed or your twins are not side-by-side, place them together. One of the magical characteristics of twins is that they have a natural ability to soothe each other.

- **Let them cry, but check on them.** It is hard to hear your baby cry, but sometimes what they need is a good cry. When you have tried everything and starting to feel overwhelmed, take a bit of a break. Set your baby down and allow them to cry. This won't harm them. They might even fall asleep. If your baby is still crying in a few minutes or after you feel better, go back in and try to calm your baby again.

- **Use soothing methods.** There are many soothing methods that you can try on your baby. For example, you can rub their back while they are in their crib, rub their little cheek, rock them, gently sing to them, or entertain them. Another struggle when it comes to soothing methods for twins is that your babies might have different methods they need at that moment.

- **Prioritize needs.** It can happen with twins often—they start crying at the same time and you are alone. The first step is not to panic. Attend to your babies calmly and see why one is crying and note what you can prioritize first. For example, if one baby is sick and the other baby is upset because their twin is sick, you will soothe your sick little one first. If one baby is crying louder than your other baby, you might tend to that one first. If you walk in the room and immediately notice one baby is crying because their pacifier fell out of their mouth, help them and then attend to your other little one.

Helping yourself cope with crying twins

You always need to remember that your mental, emotional, and physical health is important. As a mother, I know how easily this is forgotten, especially when you have upset babies. I had to slowly learn that to truly care and help my children, I needed to focus on myself first. This is a hard realization to come to as a mother because we feel selfish. But, taking care of our own health is not selfish, it is powerful as it allows us to care for our babies better.

If you need help when it comes to your babies because you feel overwhelmed by their cries— reach out for help. Here are some other tips to consider to help you deal with the crying.

- **Let go of the guilt.** As mothers, we have loads of guilt that we carry around with us on a daily basis. We feel that we don't do enough for our babies or that we aren't enough for them. We want to give them the best, but we feel like we can't. I have been there, and I know you have too. The best step to take it to work on dropping the guilt and here is why—*you are enough for your babies*. Say it out loud if you need to, "I am enough for my babies." When you feel overwhelmed, take a deep breath and keep in mind that this situation will pass, and you are doing a great job.

- **Have some "me time" every day.** It is hard to find an alone time when you have one baby, much less two or more, but it is necessary. Instead of running around trying to get all the housework done, take some time when they are sleeping for yourself. Get up a few minutes earlier and get your morning routine completed before your babies wake up.

- **It is okay to cry.** Sometimes we just need a good cry, just like our babies do. If you feel the need to cry to let out some stress or built-up emotions, go ahead and cry. Take a nice long and relaxing bath when your babies are sleeping and cry it out. You can even take time to cry yourself when your babies are crying as it might help all of you to cry it out together.

- **Remember your support system.** Talk to other moms of multiples, friends, or family members. Let them know how you are feeling. Don't keep your emotions inside as this will only cause you, and your babies, more stress.

Monitoring Your Baby's Growth

Every baby grows at a different pace, but it is important to ensure that you take your time to monitor your baby's growth so you can catch anything that does not seem right immediately. Your pediatrician will do this, but you must do it as well.

Your baby's genetics, environment, health, and activity level will play an important role in their development. It is important to note that if your baby is a little under or over the average weight or height that it is something you want to monitor, but remember it is not always bad. Your baby's doctor will help you find a solution to why they are gaining weight at a faster rate than most babies their age.

When you monitor your baby's growth, you will pay attention to these factors:

- **Weight.** To get the best weight of your baby, you will want to use a baby scale. You will normally take off their clothing to weigh them. Baby scales are used up to one year of age.

- **Length.** You will measure the length of your baby with a tape measure. You want to lay them on a table and measure them from their head to their feet.

- **Head circumference.** You can measure the head circumference to help you understand where your baby sits with their brain development. For example, if the circumference is smaller than most babies, it might signal developmental delays. If your baby has a larger than average head, they could have a medical condition known as hydrocephalus, which means they have fluid on their brain.

When you first look at a growth chart, you might think it is more confusing than it is helpful. It can be hard to understand at first, but once you have the numbers, you can use the following steps to read where your baby sits on the growth chart:

1. Decide if you are looking at your child's height or weight and note where your child fits on the side of the graph.

2. Look for your baby's age at the top of the graph.

3. Follow the lines until they meet in the graph. They will fall somewhere along the curves.

4. Once you find where the lines intersect, follow the curves so you can see the percentile where your baby sits. This percentage will show where your baby is compared to other babies their age. For

example, if your baby weighs at 9%, they are heavier than 9% of all over babies. This might indicate that they are a bit underweight and you should make sure to contact your child's primary care doctor to see what you can change to help your baby gain weight. The doctor can also make sure that your baby doesn't have a medical condition that is keeping them from gaining weight.

The key to following growth charts is to remember that it is not the specific percentage that you should be worried about. While it is helpful for doctors, they will pay more attention to the patterns your baby shows within the growth chart. For example, if they were at 7% six months ago when it came to weight and they are now at 9%, they are gaining weight. However, if the doctor sees this percentage number decreasing, they might become a little more concerned. Above all, you always want to remember that babies grow at different paces. Your baby might not have hit their growth spurt yet, while most children their age have reached the growth spurt.

Tweaking Your Toddler's Twin Routine

As your twins grow older, making sure they are on the same schedule will become a little easier. In fact, by the time they are two years old, your twins will give you a break by helping you sync up their schedules, which is nice providing they continue to keep you more than busy throughout the day.

To give you a better understanding of how eating, bathing, and sleeping work with your twin toddlers, here are some of the highs and lows to look forward to.

Eating

Your twins are about two years old and can now feed themselves for the most part. While it will get messy now and then, especially when they decide to place the noodles in their hair instead of their mouth, it eases your stress during mealtime. When it comes to drinking, you can start getting them to use cups without a lid. Some people like to allow their children to practice drinking out of "big boy" or "big girl" cups before they put any liquids in the cups. You can turn this into a little game by allowing them to have "tea time."

The biggest challenge when it comes to eating is that your twins are not the same person. What one twin likes, the other one might not. This means you might need to give them two different snacks and sometimes make two different vegetables. You do not want to force your toddler to eat the food in front of them as this will make them dread mealtime. Instead, you want to follow their lead. If they are not hungry, save the food for when they get hungry. Sometimes making food that both your toddlers will eat is a big enough challenge and you do not need to add to this challenge by having them start crying because they need to come and eat their food.

Part of their eating routine at this age is that they are trying new foods. Continue to offer your children new foods and if they do not like one type of food, wait a few weeks before you offer it again. It will be like a new food to your child because they will not remember trying it before and they might like it this time.

Bath time

If you thought babies splashed a lot in the bathtub, just wait until you place your toddlers in the tub. Sure, they can now listen to your commands of "no splashing" better than before, you can still allow them to have fun splashing and playing with toys. They are even old enough to help you wipe up all the water that they got on the floor. The best news when it comes to bath time is your twins will have the best time in the tub with each other as they play.

The challenge is that they might have too much fun, which can cause a mess in the tub. Even if you find yourself leaving the room for five seconds, you can come back to a pool on your floor. They have also learned how to team up to get into a little trouble here and there, so you need to watch out. One might be behind the curtain because they decided it is a good idea to splash you as you walk into the room. Do your best to remain calm in moments like this. Remember, they can always help you clean it up, which will help them to understand the consequences and taking responsibility.

If you find that bath time is becoming too challenging with both your twins at the same time, then you will want to look at splitting them up with back to back bath times. Of course, this might not be possible if you are a single parent. However, if you trust your toddler being in their room with the television on or playing quietly while you give the other a bath, then you can do this.

Sleeping

I will never forget getting a text from my friend at 10:30 p.m saying, "They are still talking to each other. I really wish they would fall asleep!" I smiled and found it cute, but I also understood her frustration. Your twins will love talking to each other during their bedtime. In fact, one twin might talk more and often talk to the other twin to sleep. So, while the best news is that your twins are synced with their bedtime routine, they can talk, they can get up and play, and one twin can easily keep the other twin up—and this can make for a crabby twin the next day.

The best way to handle your twins at bedtime and naptime is to let them do their little talking until they fall asleep. Usually, once one twin falls asleep the other twin will start to get bored and nod off. They might talk to themselves for a bit, but consider this their time. It is important that your twins have alone time as well. If one twin wakes up before the other twin, let that twin stay in their crib or room. This will help keep their schedules synced.

Chapter 4: Know the Reason Behind the Cry

You know that your baby has different cries to tell you what they need, but you might not completely understand all of their cries perfectly. In general, there are seven main types of cries, which are discussed below.

Seven Types of Cries

1. Hungry

The earliest stages of hunger will not involve crying. Your baby will start communicating that they are hungry by showing you cues of hunger, such as sucking on their fingers, reaching for your breast, or opening their mouth and acting like they are sucking. You will notice their tongue moving to the roof of their mouth. If you do not respond to these early signs, your baby will start to become squirmy and eventually cry. Some people refer to hunger crying as a rhythmic "neh" cry that sounds low-pitched and repetitive.

The only step you can take to soothe your baby from their hunger is the obvious one: feed them. You should feed them as soon as you notice the early stages of hunger. If you delay their feeding and your baby becomes upset it can cause them to later throw up their food.

2. Tired or uncomfortable

Even before crying, your baby will show early signs of tiredness. They may rub their eyes or face, avoid eye contact, or yawn. The earlier you catch their signs of fatigue, the easier it will be to put your baby down to sleep later. When your baby starts crying because they are tired, their cry will build with intensity. Some people refer to the cry as an "owh" sound, while other people describe the cry as nasally or whiny cry. When your baby is uncomfortable or too hot or too cold, they will have the same type of cry. But in the case of discomfort, they will give you slightly different cues. Instead of rubbing their eyes, your baby will squirm or arch themselves.

When your baby is tired, your best option is to place them down for a nap. If they are uncomfortable, start by changing their diaper and looking for signs of diaper rash. Next, think about whether your baby is chilly or too warm and if any clothing adjustments need to be made.

3. Had enough

Your baby will let you know when they have had enough. Along with a cry that sounds more like a whine, your baby will try to move away from the stimuli that are making them mad or stressed. The best option is to remove your baby from the overwhelming environment and comfort them.

4. Bored

When your baby is bored, they will try to interact with you by looking your way, smiling, cooing, or playing in their own way. For example, they might kick their legs or fiddle with their feet or hands. Their playful manner will then turn into fussing if they feel you are not giving them the attention they are craving. You will notice their fussing turning into sounds of whining or disgruntled cries. At this point, your baby is frustrated and they want to know why you aren't playing with them.

The best step to take to keep your baby from giving you their boredom cry is to take notice of their cues of boredom. Once they start interacting with you, play with them. You don't always need to go and pick them up when they are bored. You can talk to them, smile back, and make sure they have an age-appropriate toy near them to play with.

6. Colic

A baby who cries for more than three hours is defined as colic. They are inconsolable as they cry, which sounds more like a high-pitched cry or scream. Some parents feel their baby is in pain, but colic is not painful for your baby. Most babies have colic close to their bedtime. A baby as young as six weeks old to three months can have colic episodes.

It isn't easy to comfort a colicky baby, but there are many ways you can try to soothe them, such as swaddling, swinging, playing white noise, walking with them, or giving them a back rub.

7. Sick

A baby who is sick will not give a loud cry unless they are in pain. Their sick cry will sound more like a low-pitched or whimper. They will show other signs of sickness, such as pulling at their ears, having a temperature, vomiting, or diarrhea. The best step to take is to make them feel comfortable. If your baby has diarrhea, vomiting, or a high temperature you need to contact your doctor. Your baby can quickly become dehydrated when they show these symptoms and this will only make them feel worse.

Other Reasons

Flatulence or gassy baby

You can tell if your baby is having tummy trouble if they are arching their back or bringing their legs toward their torso. Their crying will start small, similar to a whimper, but it will become more intense over time. The best step is to help them get their gas moving by gently pushing their knees up toward their stomach, laying them on their right side and rubbing their left side, or giving them a back rub.

Reflux

If you notice your baby gagging or coughing when they are eating, they might have reflux. They will often spit up or vomit after they are done eating. Reflux can also cause problems when it comes to burping, which doesn't help their tummy trouble.

One of the best steps is to place your baby in an upright position, as this will help their food stay down. In fact, a baby with reflux will tend to cry when you put them in the regular feeding position because it is uncomfortable for them.

It's important to stick to your baby's feeding schedule if they have trouble with reflux because feeding them more than necessary can make their reflux worse.

Allergies

Food allergies are the most common types of allergies for a baby and can show up as hives, gastrointestinal issues, or a rash. Your baby's allergy cry will be similar to their gassy cry. They can show the same symptoms like flatulence, as this is a sign of food allergies, making it hard to distinguish between gas and allergies. If your baby recently tried a new type of food, such as milk, fish, or wheat, you need to discuss this with your doctor at your baby's next checkup.

Other types of allergies that can affect your baby are seasonal and medical allergies. For seasonal allergies, your baby will have watery eyes, a runny nose, and a cough. It might seem like they have a cold at first, but you will notice the symptoms continuing or only showing up with certain environmental factors, such as rain.

The only way to truly know if your baby has allergies is through an allergy test, which their doctor can perform. The best step you can take is to keep a journal of your baby's allergies. Be sure to write down their symptoms, what they ate, and any environmental factors that could contribute to the allergy.

When You Can't Find a Reason for the Crying

Sometimes babies do not have a reason for their crying session. In fact, sometimes babies who cry for a few minutes to an hour have no reason at all. This type of crying moment tends to happen in the evening, which makes many people feel it is because their baby is tired or overstimulated. This can also be one of the most stressful times of the day as everyone is trying to get their evening routine done so they can go to bed as everyone is tired. In these moments, the best step you can take is to allow your baby to have their crying moment and try to comfort them if they can't calm down.

Learn to Understand Your Baby's Cry

Don't worry if you feel overwhelmed thinking that you will never learn your baby's specific cries because *you will*. You will quickly catch on to your baby's form of communication and be able to help them quickly. Once you understand your baby's cries, you will find that they cry less often and seem to coo a bit more. Before you know it, they will be learning how to talk! So, even if you feel stressed about your baby's cries now, know that they will be a thing of the past one day. Do your best to enjoy your moments by noting the different cries and learning how to effectively communicate with your baby. Doing this will only make your bond grow stronger.

Another key is to stick to the routine. Your baby needs a routine and they can become frustrated or uncomfortable when their routine is not in place. You might not think they know, but they do. Sticking to a routine can also help you identify the cries. For example, if it is close to bedtime and your baby starts crying, they might be saying they are tired now and are ready for bed.

Surviving the Crying Spells

Every baby has crying spells. No matter what you try to calm your baby's cries, sometimes it is just not what they need because they are simply inconsolable. These moments are upsetting and cause a lot of anxiety for the parent(s). While the crying won't harm your baby, it can leave you feeling like you are not enough. Studies have proven that these moments can create emotional, mental, and physical effects on parents.

The best step you can do is to take care of yourself as well. This is not always easy to do, and I know it is easier said than done, but it is necessary to do what you can to ease your anxiety and pain. Here are a few tips to help you through the process.

- **Stay healthy.** Make sure that you get all the sleep you can, take care of yourself by eating right and exercising. Ensure you allow yourself some "me time" and you will find yourself able to care for your baby more easily, even though their crying spells.

- **Breathe.** Take a few deep breaths and remember that the crying spell will not last forever.

- **Understand your own limits.** Everyone has limits. This does not make you a bad parent just because you need to ask for help or are afraid you will lose control if your baby does not stop crying. Every parent goes through this. All you need to do is place your child down and let them cry for a few minutes so you can calm yourself down. Never hesitate to reach out for help or moral support if you need it.

- **Take a break.** Do not be afraid to tell a friend, your partner, or a family member that you need to take a bit of a break. Ask them to come over and help care for the baby. Even if it is just so you can take a nap or go for a walk, it will help you and your baby in the end.

Chapter 5: A Parent's Biggest Fear

For some parents, sleep training makes them feel guilty, especially if they are using a cry it out method. They also fear that their baby will remember them not going in their room right away to check on them or help them back to sleep. While guilt and fear are understandable, they are not realistic. Part of this is the belief that the cry it out method means you do not go in to check on your baby. This is not the cry it out method at all. You set a certain amount of time where you allow your baby to fuss or cry to see if they will soothe themselves back to sleep. If they do not do this by the timeframe you gave yourself, such as two minutes, then you go in and soothe them to sleep.

The biggest fear parents have is that they will harm their baby, one way or another, by using any sleep training method. A *Pediatrics* study aims to end this fear by stating that you will not harm your baby by using any of the sleep methods, whether you focus on a no tears method or a cry it out method. You will help your child get the sleep they need and live a happy and healthy life by getting them to follow a sleeping schedule.

In this study, 43 babies between the ages of six to 16 months were placed in one of three groups. The first group used the graduated extension method which tells parents to periodically check on their baby. The second group used bedtime fading, which focuses on gradually delaying the baby's bedtime as a way to introduce sleepiness. The third group is known as the control group and only received information about the best sleep practices they could incorporate (Ruiz, 2016).

The study concluded that the first group, which used a cry it out method, did not affect their babies negatively in any way. The bonds between the parents and babies remained strong, which is something that many people felt would not be proven by this study. At the time of this study, most people felt that any type of cry it out method caused the babies to resent their parents because they did not receive what they needed. The researchers further tested the stress hormone of the baby measuring their cortisone levels. They found no difference in the stress level because of the sleep training method used (Ruiz, 2016).

This is not the only study completed to show that babies have no long-term effects when it comes to the cry it out method. There are several studies that give us the same result, telling parents that there is no reason to fear the cry it out method. You do not need to worry about damaging the bond you have with your little one to make sure they get a good night's sleep.

The studies are also here to tell you to let go of the guilt. I know this is easier said than done, but there is no reason to feel guilty about letting your baby cry for a couple of minutes before you go in to help soothe them. You are raising an independent child, and this is something you need to be proud of. Your baby will continue to grow up to know that you love them and are there for them when they need you. At the same time, they will learn how to self-soothe themselves to sleep, get a good night's rest, and allow everyone else in the household to do the same. This will keep you happy, which will also keep your baby happy and thriving.

What Science Cannot Tell Us About the Cry It Out Method

Even though there are a number of studies to support, and some that do not, the cry it out method, there are several factors that science cannot tell us. To help you understand the cry it out method a little better, we will go through myths and then state the facts about the method. From there, we can come up with our own conclusion and you can have a better idea when it comes to deciding which sleep training method you will use.

Myth: The only sleep training method you can use is the cry it out method.

Fact: There are many different sleep training methods that parents and experts feel are great methods. Some of these methods are a cry it out method while others are not. Furthermore, people continue to create their own sleep training methods that work for their babies and share them with the rest of the world.

Myth: You need to find the correct amount of time to let your baby cry while you are sleep training. You do not want to go over or under this amount of time.

Fact: You need to follow your instincts and there is no set "right" time when it comes to letting your baby cry during sleep training. Some people will wait a minute while other parents will wait three minutes. The ones who wait longer are just as good of parents as the parents who wait a minute. The amount of time you allow your child to cry does not indicate if you are a good parent or not. There is no right or wrong formula when it comes to sleep training and crying. You need to do what is best for you and what feels right for your baby.

Myth: Sleep training will hurt my baby in the long run.

Fact: As you can see from the study above, sleep training will not harm your baby. Your baby will get the sleep they need and begin to thrive even more with sleep training.

Myth: The only way to truly know that you are sleep training is when you hear a lot of crying.

Fact: While you can use this as a way to know that sleep training is working, there are several approaches that many people feel are gentler. You always want to remember to use what is best for you and what you feel is best for your baby. This means that you do not let other people tell you how sleep training between you and your baby should go. You can get advice, but you always need to follow your instincts and your heart. You need to be comfortable with sleep training, so your baby has a calm environment. You will know it is working when they start to sleep on their schedule and sleep for longer periods of time.

Myth: Once my baby is sleep trained, they will not wake up during the night and I can get a full night's sleep.

Fact: It is natural for babies to wake up a few times during the night, even if they are sleep trained. This is very common within their first year of life. The key to sleep training is you help your baby learn to self-soothe themselves back to sleep. Yes, they will wake up fewer times, which means you will wake up less, but they will still wake up from time to time.

Conclusion

Looking at the myths and facts when it comes to sleep training your baby, it is important to note that it is helpful for the whole family. Not only will your baby get enough sleep, but you will too. Furthermore, sleep training can help your baby thrive, which will support them on their road to healthy development.

Chapter 6: Why Most Training Fails

The Top 10 Reasons Sleep Training Fails

Sleep training does not fail simply because you didn't or couldn't accomplish the task. It fails because of the common mistakes that most parents make. Here are some of the most common mistakes to be aware of and work to avoid in the sleep training process.

1. Starting sleep training at the wrong time

The best time to start sleep training is when your baby understands the difference between day and night and are on their own sleep cycle. The first sign your baby is on their sleep cycle if they sleep and stay awake for a predictable period of time. For example, you might notice your baby sleeping for 90 minutes and then waking up for about 30 minutes. After noticing this schedule for a few days, you can start looking at a sleep training plan.

If you are trying to sleep train a toddler, you should stay away from starting the sleep training at the same time as other milestone moments, such as potty training. These moments naturally interfere with your child's sleep schedule and will cause the sleep training process to fail.

2. Not changing the bedtime

To ensure that sleep training is successful, you need to start at a certain time and stick to it. If you have a bedtime that is too early, your child will not be tired enough to sleep. Many people state it is best to have a bedtime that is a little later as you want to lay them down when they are about to fall asleep, yet still awake. Furthermore, it is best to keep the bedtime routine under 30 minutes and to stick with the routine. This means, especially as your child gets older, it is only one book and not two one night and then one the next night. You also want to read for the same amount of time every night.

3. Missing the medical causes of sleep difficulties

Earlier, I mentioned the importance of seeing your baby's primary care doctor before you start sleep training. Following this step will help you learn if your baby is ready for sleep training and make sure that they do not have a medical issue to keep them from successful sleep training. Sleep issues do not mean you can't sleep train your baby. It simply means that you will work with the doctor to manage these issues before you begin the sleep training process.

4. Being inconsistent

You have a busy life. You are tired after work or when it gets to be bedtime. You lose energy, which makes you question whether you have to go through the sleep training process or if you can skip it for that night. Many times, people will skip part of the process or won't follow through with their timing because they are exhausted. While this is understandable, and nothing to feel guilty about, it can cause your sleep training to fail.

Do your best to push through when you are tired. Stick to your sleep training plan as the most important part of this process is that your baby has a consistent schedule to learn. If you find yourself needing help for a couple of nights, reach out and ask a friend or family member to help you. Allow yourself to go to bed early and get up with your baby. This can help you stay consistent.

5. Challenges in the bedroom

There are several challenges that can show themselves when it comes to sleep training and some of them you might not think about. For example, if you live on a noisy street, you might not notice how the noise keeps your baby up or wakes them up as they are about to fall asleep.

Another common challenge is a sibling in the same room as your baby. If this is the case, the best method is to move the other child into your bedroom, a spare bedroom, or even the couch during sleep training.

Other challenges include light, even street lights. Lights that shine directly on your child can keep them awake. If you can read in your child's room, especially in the spot where they are sleeping, the light is too bright for them. Get blinds to block out any outside light or find a light for them that has a dimmer switch.

6. Not being ready

Sometimes parents start sleep training their baby too early. Sleep training is not a task that you can wake up one morning and decide you will start this process that night. You need to prepare yourself and your baby for the sleep training journey. This means that you will want to set a start date. You want to have your plan, method, and everything in place by the time your start date comes. This includes a doctor's visit and making sure any helpers understand and support the plan.

7. Moving your child into their bedroom at the same time

You want to make sure your baby is comfortable sleeping in their own room before you start sleep training. If you start the process at the same time you move them into their own bedroom, your child will feel too much stress as this is too much change all at once. You need to work with them and introduce change slowly into their life. You don't need to move your child into their room months before you start sleep training. It usually only takes a few nights to a week for your child to become comfortable with their new sleeping environment.

8. Feeding your child all night long

Instead of feeding your child several times during the night when you start the sleep training process, many experts state you should feed them right before bed. When you first start, even if it is at six months of age, you will still need to wake up at least once during the night to feed your baby. This is fine. You can still sleep train your child as you feed them once or twice during the night. However, waking them up multiple times or having them wake up several times to eat is not something that will help sleep training.

9. The "extinction burst"

The "extinction burst" means your baby's crying or certain behavior will get worse before it gets better. For example, you place your baby into their crib and follow the "cry it out" method. You feel pleased because the first night went better than you thought. However, the second night was the opposite. Your baby cried for over an hour. While you checked on them every 10 minutes and tried to soothe them, they would start screaming once you left the room. After the second night of this, you felt like a failure with sleep training because it seemed to get worse and not better.

The fact is, you need to hold on. It can take up to a week for sleep training to work with your baby. If it is longer than a week and you do not see any signs of improvement, you should contact your baby's pediatrician and make sure there are no underlying medical issues.

10. Switching to a bed prematurely

Most experts state you should not switch your baby to a toddler bed until they are about two years old. There are a few exceptions, such as climbing out of the crib. One mistake you can make when it comes to sleep training is switching your baby to a toddler bed and then starting the sleep training process. Your baby always needs to be comfortable in their sleeping environment before you start the sleep training process.

Misguided Approaches to Sleep Training (How to Troubleshoot Sleep Training)

The number one reason

The number one reason why sleep training fails is that people expect their babies to learn quickly. One reason for this is because there are many people who say their child learned within a few days and many experts who state babies should adjust to their schedules within a week.

The reality is, your baby is on their own time frame and they might take longer than a week to adjust. You want to make sure that your expectations of sleep training are realistic. If you have unrealistic expectations, you will create extra stress when it comes to sleep training. This will make sleep training harder for both you and your baby as the atmosphere will not be calming. To help your baby sleep, you want to create a calm and warm environment.

The key to sleep training is to remember that you are your baby's teacher. You are helping them learn a new skill—that they can soothe themselves to sleep. Many parents will give up on a task after the first night or two if they do not feel that it is working. You should always try the same schedule at least three nights in a row. If you find on the fourth night that the process is not becoming easier, consider looking at your sleep training plan and see where you can adjust. Is there something that causes your baby to become anxious? Did you start too early? Are you using a method that works for you and your baby? Do you put them to bed too late or too early? There are many factors to consider, but you are bound to find one that causes you to go, "ah, this might be the problem" and adjust your sleep training plan.

What is missing?

The biggest factor that is missing when it comes to sleep training is consistency. It is hard to remain consistent every day as your life is not always meant to follow a consistent path. However, you always need to do what you can when it comes to your baby. This means you might need to tell your friends that you cannot stay out beyond 6:30, but you need to get home to start putting your baby to bed. It means that you will need to push through your baby's bedtime routine when you are exhausted and feel that you can hardly function yourself.

If you naturally struggle with consistency, try to find an accountability buddy. This is someone, such as your friend, partner, or family member that can help you keep on schedule. They do not need to live with you, they can simply call you and make sure that you are starting the bedtime routine and staying on track. If you are struggling, they might come and help you that night or talk you through any challenges that you are experiencing.

Chapter 7: What Sleep Method is Right for My Baby? (Choose a Sleep Method That Works for Your Family)

Oh, the big question when it comes to sleep training, "Which sleep method is right for my baby and my family?" This question is always harder for people who have other young children in the home or single parents who know they will need to go through the whole process by themselves. For parent(s) with other children, they need to find something that will work for them too and this can cause other problems, especially if their baby sleeps in the same room with another sibling. A single parent will wonder what method they will emotionally and psychologically be able to handle consistently.

How Do I Pick the Right Method for Me and for My Baby?

The bottom line is, you need to focus on you and not just your baby and your family members. All sleep training methods allow you to modify your baby's behavior, so they learn to self-soothe themselves to sleep. If you will be the primary person to follow through on the sleep training process, you need to ensure that you can emotionally, mentally, and physically handle the sleep training method or you will struggle to remain consistent. You might stop trying to train your baby to self-soothe themselves to sleep after a couple of nights because you feel it is too hard. For example, if you know you cannot tolerate hearing your baby cry themselves to sleep, even when you go in their bedroom and help soothe them, the "cry it out" method might not be a suitable choice for you.

You need to choose a method that you are comfortable with because your baby will feel what you feel. If you feel uncomfortable about the method, they will more likely feel uncomfortable. This will cause them to struggle when it comes to learning the sleep training method and you will quickly deem it as a failure.

There are a lot of factors you will look at when you choose a method. Some methods you will read about and automatically know they are not the right fit for you and your baby. Other methods you will research deeply, and you might make a pros and cons list that helps you decide which method is the best. Your personality, age, baby's patterns, and personal beliefs will all come into your decision-making process.

The best advice that you can receive when it comes to picking a method is to follow your intuition. If a method doesn't feel right to you, don't use that method. There are a lot of great methods available to you and one will feel like the perfect fit for your family.

If you have a partner or are co-parenting, you do not want to leave them out of the decision-making process. Even if you are the primary parent and will do most of the sleep training, the system will only work if both parents are on board. If your partner does not agree with the method, they might not care to follow through and remain consistent, which will affect the baby more than anyone else.

Sleep Training Methods

Cry It Out Method

Contrary to popular belief, the cry it out method does not state that you need to let your baby cry in their crib until they fall asleep. The method states that you will set a period of time that you let your baby cry before you go in to comfort them. There are many different versions of this method and you will tweak it to create a strategy that works best for you, your baby, and anyone else involved.

Richard Ferber, a pediatrician, is credited with developing the main idea behind the cry it out method. While he never coined the phrase "cry it out" he supported parents allowing their babies a period to cry it out during sleep training because he felt you cannot avoid this part of sleep training.

The main theory behind the cry it out method is that if you continue to soothe your baby to sleep by rocking them or rubbing their back, you cannot teach them to fall asleep on their own. They will constantly want you to soothe them to sleep. It is important to note that crying is not the goal when it comes to this method. It is simply a part of the method. The goal is the same as any other sleep training strategy—to teach your baby to put themselves to sleep when they are supposed to and sleep throughout the night.

Jodi Mindell follows much of Ferber's "cry it out" method but is considered to be gentler. She focuses on giving her patients a variety of tips to follow to help their baby learn to self-soothe instead of parents focusing strictly on sleep training. She uses experiences from her job of treating sleep problems to help parents find the best technique within the cry it out method that works for them.

Michel Cohen is a pediatrician who supports the cry it out method. Cohen believes that you can start sleep training babies as young as eight weeks old by letting them cry for a period of time.

If you want to try one of the cry it out methods, you should follow these basic steps. Remember, you also need to pay attention to your baby's cues and how well you can handle the method. Follow your instincts for the best outcome.

1. Talk to your baby's pediatrician about when you should start sleep training your baby. They should be between the age of four to six months, but it also depends on other factors, such as if they were premature.

2. Set a start date and make sure you have a plan. Know how long you will let your baby cry it out. For example, you might start with two minutes and slowly increase the length of time.

3. While your baby is drowsy but still awake, place them in their crib.

4. Tell your baby goodnight and leave the room. If your baby starts to cry, wait until your set time is up to walk back into the room.

5. Soothe your baby by patting or rubbing them on their back for about a minute or until they are calmer.

6. Walk back out of the room. If your baby starts crying again, wait until a little longer than the first time. For example, if you waited two minutes the first time, you can wait three minutes the next time.

7. Follow this routine until your child falls asleep.

8. If your child wakes up during the night, repeat the routine until they are asleep.

Along with a routine, there are many tips that you can use when trying a cry it out method.

- **Realize there will be a few tough nights.** It will take time for your baby to adjust to their new routine, which means you will need to sit through a few difficult nights of listening to your baby cry and going into their room several times to soothe them. Some parents state it took them close to three weeks while other parents say it was about a week.

- **Know that you will lose some sleep.** The first night will be the hardest and you want to make sure that you start on a night where you can lose a good amount of sleep. For example, if you work Monday through Friday, you will want to start on a Friday night as you will be able to get more sleep come Sunday night.

- **Relapses will happen.** Even when your child has started to self-soothe themselves to sleep, they will relapse occasionally. This is bound to happen when you take a family vacation, they are sleeping in a different house, or they are not feeling well.

If you are comfortable with the cry it out method and you are consistent, it will work well for you, your baby, and everyone else involved. However, if you are at your wit's end and there is no sign of the crying lightening up, you will want to look at a different method.

One parent who tried the cry it out method stated that after trying several methods, she finally decided to try the cry it out method when her daughter turned seven months old. While it took nearly four weeks, her baby continues to sleep well and she credits this method.

Another mother supports the cry it out method and it worked within the first night. Not only did her baby sleep all night after self-soothing themselves to sleep, but they slept about 12 hours the following night.

The main reason why people are against the cry it out method is that they feel it is more stressful for their baby—and themselves. While it is hard for parent(s) to hear their baby cry and not try to soothe them immediately, it is not more stressful for the baby unless you leave them to cry for too long. Babies will become overwhelmed when they are crying and are not cared for by a certain period of time. They can become so upset that they vomit, which is why you want to set a time by following your baby's personality and stick with that time. You can slowly start to increase your time as your baby starts to calm down and begins to soothe themselves.

No Tears Method

There are many reasons why people look at the no tears method. One reason is that parents know they cannot stand to hear their baby cry alone. Another reason is that they tried another method, such as the cry it out method, and it did not work for them.

Most parents who follow the no tears method use bedtime as a way to bond with their baby. This method allows them to develop a bedtime routine that is quiet and calm as these factors will help your baby drift into a peaceful sleep. When your baby falls asleep in this manner, they are less likely to wake up during the night. When they do wake up or if they have a difficult time falling asleep, you respond to them. You feed them if they give you the cry of hunger and comfort them if they are not content with their environment.

The no tears method seems to be the opposite of the cry it out method. Many people feel if you support the no tears method, then you do not support the cry it out method. While this is not completely true, most experts will agree with either the cry it out or the no tears method.

Experts who support the no tears method state that it is more soothing for the baby. They are less likely to feel overwhelmed and will start to trust that their parent(s) will take care of them when they cry out. The no-cry method will help make babies feel well-adjusted. Experts who support the cry it out method state that the no tears method will make babies become overly dependent on their parent(s). They will not learn how to independently put themselves to sleep.

There are a number of experts who discuss the no tears method.

- William Sears is a pediatrician who supports the no tears method and often discusses this method with his patients. To help them through their sleep training phase, William uses his personal experiences guide parents through sleep training. He doesn't believe in a "one size fits all" sleep method. Instead, he says to focus on your family maintaining closeness with your baby by following their cues in order to develop the best sleep training approach for the whole family.

- Parent educator Elizabeth Pantly tells parents that they need to help soothe their baby to sleep so they can learn to self-soothe. For example, you can rock your baby and sing them a quiet and soothing lullaby until they are sleepy. Once they get to this point, you then gently lay them down in their bed and leave the room or back away. When your baby starts to fuss or cry, you tend to them immediately and continue to soothe them to a state of drowsiness.

- Tracy Hogg, a nurse, follows most aspects of the no tears method but does not agree with certain forms of soothing, such as patting or rubbing your baby's back. She believes that babies can become dependent on this type of soothing and it won't help them learn to self-soothe. Instead, they will feel the need to have you rub their backs when they are unable to fall asleep. Hogg states that parents should pick their baby up when they are crying and then place them back down. You should repeat these steps until your baby stops crying or falls asleep.

One of the factors about the no tears method is you can use your own soothing techniques and not follow a specific set of steps. For example, you might disagree with Hogg that you should not rub your baby's back until they fall asleep. Instead, you pick them up, hold them until they calm down, and then lay them back down. Even if you repeat these steps 20 times within an hour, it is what you believe is right for everyone involved.

Even though you do not need to follow every step, there are several practical tips that can help you develop your no tears method.

- **Ensure all changes to your baby's routine are gradual.** No matter what part of your baby's routine you are focusing on changing, you need to make sure they are not too sudden. Your baby can tell when their routine is changing so if you change the routines quickly, they won't feel comfortable and can become fussy. For example, if you are changing their feeding time because you don't want your baby to fall asleep as you feed them, you should move the time by five minutes every few days. If you normally feed your baby about 7:00 p.m. and they fall asleep by 7:10, you might decide to start feeding them at 6:55 p.m. After a couple of days, you can change the time to 6:50 and then finally 6:45 p.m., a time that ensures that your baby will still be awake when you finish feeding.

- **If your baby is sleepy, put them to bed a little early.** Your baby will have days where they are more tired than normal, just like you. On these days, you will start to notice your baby showing the cues that they are ready for bed, such as rubbing their eyes and face. Even if it is 30 minutes before your baby usually goes to bed, it is perfectly fine to start their bedtime routine sooner. If you don't do this, your baby can quickly become overtired, which can make it harder for them to fall and stay asleep.

- **Develop keywords to use during bedtime.** Even though your baby cannot verbally communicate words with you, you can still communicate verbally with them. To ensure they understand what you are telling them, you want to use keywords, such as "ssshhh" or "mommy's here." Using keywords during their bedtime routine will let them know that it is time to go to bed. Furthermore, it will allow you to bond with your baby is a specific way and give them the comfort that you are there with them.

- **Ensure your baby is comfortable in their sleeping area.** You will start to notice your baby's personality when you are in the hospital. In fact, some people begin to feel parts of their personality when they are still in the womb. You want to follow your baby's personality when creating their sleeping area so it's as comfortable and calming as possible for them. For example, if your baby likes to fall asleep by watching colorful lights, make sure that you have lights that your baby can look at during the night. When they wake up in the middle of the night, they will notice the lights and this will help them soothe themselves back to sleep. If your baby likes a stuffed bear, place the bear up on a shelf where they can see the toy as this can help soothe them to sleep as well.

- **Don't jump up at every sound you hear coming from your child's bedroom.** It is normal for your baby to make a little whimper sound now and then. They might make this sound when they are in a half asleep and half awake state or even when they are still sleeping. If you hear a noise coming from your baby, wait a minute to see if they actually start crying and need you to come in to help them fall back asleep.

While no tears method works in time, it will not work for every baby. If this method is to work for your baby, you need to have patience as it will take a while for your baby to learn to self-soothe themselves to sleep. It is true that the cry it out method does not take as long. However, many people believe that no tears method is less traumatic for your baby in the long run, which makes this method work better for some.

Parents who have tried the no tears approach and stated that it worked, give the following tips:

- **Be patient.** You will have nights where you feel like you are picking up your baby 100 times and it seemingly will never end. You will also have nights when they go down a little easier. The number of times you pick up your baby might gradually decrease before they learn to self-soothe themselves to sleep. You can also notice the number of times you need to pick up your baby increases after it decreased for a few nights. No matter what happens, you need to remain consistent and not give up.

- **Co-sleeping works.** Some mothers talk about how their babies learned to fall asleep within a couple of nights because they co-slept with their baby. Once the mothers felt their baby squirming in the bed or heard them make a noise, they fed their babies and noticed them falling back asleep quickly. In fact, many mothers agreed that their babies didn't even fully wake up to eat.

- **Soothe your baby to sleep without taking them out of the crib.** Many parents discuss how they will rock their babies to sleep but won't pick them up once they lay down. Instead, they will rub their stomach, arm, or hum gently. They feel taking their baby out of the crib can wake them up more. It is easier for your baby to learn it is time to sleep when they remain in the bed.

Chapter 8: Good Nights Start With Good Days

Why Is It So Hard to Get on a Schedule?

From the moment your baby comes into this world, you will want to start focusing on a schedule. It will take a while for your newborn to adapt to their schedule, but they will soon find peace.

The Order of Events in Your Baby's Day

Your newborn will have a different order of events than an older baby. For instance, when it comes to newborns, they have three major events that happen throughout their day:

1. Feeding

2. Changing their diaper

3. Sleeping

When you are developing a schedule with your newborn, you want to try to follow this sequence of events around the same time every day. For instance, your newborn eats every three hours, so you will start the routine by scheduling their feeding time every third hour. After feeding time, you burp them and interact with them a bit before changing their diaper. At this point, it is time for them to sleep.

You have probably heard about the eat-sleep-play routine. While most people will tell you it works like a charm, it does not work for everyone. One reason this routine does not work for every baby is that babies are individuals. One routine will work for one child but not the next. Another reason the routine does not work, specifically for breastfed babies is because they work on a supply and demand basis with you. Furthermore, breastfeeding gives your baby a special bond with you that is more important than placing them in a certain routine. The

138

bottom line is you need to find a routine that works for you and your baby.

Nap Training

Some experts will tell you that you need to follow your bedtime routine when it comes to naptime. Other experts will tell you that you need to create a new routine for naptime so your baby understands the difference between bedtime and naptime. Of course, you need to do what is best for you and your baby. If this means you sing them a lullaby as you do when they go to bed, by all means, sing!

When it comes to nap training, you want to wait until your baby is about three to four months old. Whether you start nap training and bedtime training at the same time is up to you. You can do one at a time, which is a great idea if your baby is struggling with sleep training, or you can start them both at the same time.

You also should know the amount of sleep your child needs for their age when you are thinking about nap training. You need to follow the daily guide for routines and do your best to make sure your child gets enough sleep throughout their day.

If you have a baby who does not care for naps, the best step to take is to create a quiet routine before naptime. You will want to do this with all babies, but it is more important for babies who fight you when it comes to their naptime. Creating a calming routine will help them become sleepy.

Effective Ways to Train Your Baby for Self-Soothing

Self-soothing allows your baby to put themselves to sleep through their own comforting techniques. They might look around at a light in their room, play with their hands, or simply lay there until they fall asleep with their eyes closed. Other forms of self-soothing involve rubbing their eyes, sucking on a blanket, toy, or pacifier, and holding their hands together like they are in prayer.

While there is no specific age when it comes to teaching your baby to soothe themselves to sleep, babies are generally not able to do this before three months of age. Usually, parents start to teach their babies to self-soothe when they start sleep training.

Around four months of age, the brain can handle the baby's emotions a bit better and they start developing their sleep pattern, which helps them become drowsy enough to use self-soothing techniques to get to sleep.

Parents like to teach their children how to soothe themselves because it holds many benefits:

- Your baby will sleep better for longer periods of time.

- As a mother, you can have a bit more time for yourself.

- Your baby will become more self-reliant.

141

- Your baby will grow up and can manage their tantrums a little better.

After reading these benefits, it is no wonder why you want to teach your child to soothe themselves to sleep. To do this, there are a few steps you need to follow.

1. If you need to change your mindset to let go of the guilt of not comforting your baby every time they fuss or cry, this is the first step you need to take. It might take time but know that you are helping your baby by teaching them how to self-soothe.

2. Make sure you set a routine for your child's 24-hours. You can use the daily guides that are placed in chapter 10 to help you establish a routine depending on your baby's age.

3. Set a time limit that will tell you when you can go into the room and comfort your baby. You can start with one minute and

slowly increase the time as they learn to self-soothe.

4. Always place your baby in bed when they are drowsy, but not sleeping.

5. Do not feed your baby to sleep.

There are a number of tips you can use to help your baby self-soothe.

- Place a musical toy next to their bed. Once they are old enough they will learn to push the button or you can turn it on and leave it for the night.

- Create a night routine that involves relaxation.

- Make sure you are consistent with their bedtime and routine.

There are many dos and don'ts that you want to follow as you help teach your baby to self-soothe.

- Always have patience. It will take time for your baby to learn their self-soothing techniques.

- While this might be difficult, you need to make sure you don't allow them to always be dependent on you putting them to sleep. This means you cannot rock them to sleep.

- Do not feed your baby to sleep. You want to separate feeding and sleeping times.

While you will not start sleep training your newborn, it is important to keep them on a schedule as this will help them develop their self-soothing skills, which are needed when it comes to sleep training. Some babies will catch on to self-soothing techniques a little quicker than others. As long as you have patience and remain consistent, your baby will gradually learn to self-soothe.

One of the biggest problems when it comes to struggling to self-soothe is babies are used to nursing before bed. If this is the case, you want to gradually push back the time you nurse your baby. You might do this by feeding them 10 minutes earlier once a week until you have separated feeding and bedtime.

To recap, here are some guidelines that you need to remember when you are self-soothing:

1. You always need to work with your baby when they are learning a new skill. This means you will practice with them until they start to understand the concept and they can do it on their own.

2. Your baby can only learn to soothe themselves to sleep when you place them in the bed while they are still awake but tired.

3. Always have patience and realize you need to go at your baby's pace and not your pace.

Chapter 9: The (Not So) Dreaded Night Training

Parents usually dread sleep training for many reasons. They may have heard that it works, but they have also heard that it means you will get less sleep for a couple of nights and that you might not find the best sleep training method right away. In other words, you might start to use one of the cry it out methods only to start on a no tears method a week later. It is true that sleep training can be exhausting. But, it is also true that when you find a method that works, it is 100% worth every moment.

What Is Sleeping Through the Night?

Sleep matures over your baby's first year, but this does not mean you need to wait a year to start sleeping through the night. But, it *does* mean you need to understand what sleeping through the night for your baby truly means.

First, your baby will not sleep through the night without waking up for a minute or a bit more. Even after you successfully sleep training your baby, they will most likely self-soothe themselves back to sleep. While they wake up, they might not fully wake up, which will allow them to easily drift back into a peaceful sleep. However, it is still important to remember that not all babies can self-soothe by six to eight months old. About 30 to 40% of babies still need help getting back to sleep when they wake up (What 'sleeping through the night' actually means, 2018).

Bedtime

When your baby is ready to sleep through the night, they will give you the following clues.

1. Your baby can put themselves back to sleep when they wake up. They might make a little whining noise or fuss for a

bit, but they will self-soothe themselves within a few minutes.

2. Your baby will sleep for longer periods of time without waking up. This usually happens around the three to the four-month mark.

3. Your baby can lay in their crib for six to eight hours without needing to call you to help them get back to sleep.

The following general guidelines vary by age group when it comes to your baby's first year.

- **Birth to six weeks.** Your baby will have between six to eight regularly occurring sleep periods. Each period will last about two to four hours. This is a 24-hour cycle, which is why it is important to get your baby on a daily schedule. Until about four weeks old, your baby does not have a day and night pattern.

- **Six weeks to three months.** Your baby's sleep time per period will increase to about four to five hours. They will continue to briefly wake up one to three times while they are sleeping during the night. This is around the time they start to learn to self-soothe themselves.

- **Three to six months.** The length of time your baby will sleep during the night in one stretch continues to increase. They are now between five to six-hour stretches, can self-soothe themselves, but might still need help getting back to sleep from time to time. Your baby will still wake up between one to three times during their nightly stretches.

- **Six to 12 months.** Your baby is still sleeping for about 12 hours during the night, but it is split into two stretches. With the proper guidance, they will self-soothe themselves to sleep during their one to three awakenings per stretch of sleep. While your baby can put themselves to sleep, they will need you to help them now and then.

- **From 12 months.** Around 12 months you will start to see your baby truly sleep through the night. They will no longer need two stretches to sleep 12 hours, but only one. They might still wake up from time to time, but it won't be an every night situation and if they do, they can usually self-soothe themselves back to sleep.

Dream feeding

Dream feeding happens when you decide to gently feed your baby before you go to bed so they will sleep longer. You do not fully wake your baby up. Instead, you just get them to eat while they are kind of in the half asleep and half awake mode. The best time to dream feed your baby is between 10:00 p.m. and midnight.

Dream feeding is a lot easier than it sounds. Many parents worry about dream feeding because they do not want to wake their babies. By following these three easy steps, you can quickly dream feed your baby without bringing them into a fully awake state.

1. Between 10:00 p.m. and midnight, around the time you are going to bed, you want to gently wake your baby from their crib.

2. Set your baby's bottle or your breast on your baby's lower lip. They should start automatically feeding without waking up.

3. Nurse for about five to 10 minutes on each side. You might have to encourage your baby to continue eating if they stop sucking.

There is a possibility that your baby will be really tired and not want to eat much, but you should still try to encourage it as much as possible. You can also tickle their toes a bit to change their diaper if they are too tired to rouse from their sleep during this time.

Remember you will want to burp your baby before you lay them back down after they dream feed. If you do not do this, you can cause them to have gas pains, which will keep your baby and you up most of the night.

Depending on your baby's age, the best step to take to get them back to sleep is to swaddle them. If your baby doesn't like swaddling, then you can simply play some low white noise or lullabies that usually put them back to sleep. If you are sleep training, you should follow your method as you always need to be consistent.

There are many benefits to dream feeding your infant:

- The meal is at a convenient time for you as it allows you to get more sleep during the night.

- Because your baby ate before she went to bed, they will not wake up due to hunger earlier in the night. They might wait two to three hours, depending on their age and their feeding schedule.

- The dream feeding gives your baby more calories, which is one reason they will sleep better.

- You do not respond to your baby's cries by feeding them. When your baby cries and you feed them, they tend to wake up and cry more during the night to eat.

If your baby wakes up around 3:00 a.m. on a regular schedule to eat, set your alarm clock for 2:30 a.m. and do another dream feed. The point of dream feeding is to feed your baby before they wake up.

When you dream feed for a second time, you want to make sure you do not give your baby the same amount of milk. For example, if you are nursing, let them eat on one side. Giving them the same amount of milk as before can cause them to have tummy trouble.

There is no specific age to stop dream feeding your baby. You want to get them to the point where they will not wake up to eat, which means you and your baby are sleeping through the night.

What if my baby wakes up during the night?

There are many steps you can take when your baby wakes up during the night. The key to remember is that you want to remain consistent with your sleep training and do what works best for you and your baby.

Your baby can wake up for many reasons during the night, such as teething, dreaming, hunger, feeling unwell, or a variety of other disturbances. Depending on why your baby wakes up might depend on how you get them back to sleep. For example, if your baby is hungry, you will give them a bottle. If your baby is teething, you will need to use another method to ease their pain, such as giving them teething medicine or a teething ring.

Another solution you can use is calm music such as lullabies or white noise. This is helpful if you live in a city where outside noise can wake your baby up. While babies can sleep deeply, their sleep cycles are very short, meaning your baby will sleep deeply for 45 minutes out of the 90 minutes they are sleeping. It's easier for your baby to wake up during the 45 minutes when they are not in a deep sleep.

Some parents like to place their hand on their baby's chest to help them fall asleep. This gives your baby the added comfort that you are still with them even when their eyes are closed.

Every baby will go through a period of separation anxiety, which usually happens around the age of six months. Separation anxiety is another reason for nightly wakings. Even if you have already successfully sleep trained your baby, they can wake up and worry because they do not see you, making it harder for them to self-soothe. If your baby is struggling with separation anxiety, go into their room and talk to them gently. Let them know that you are there, but try to refrain from picking them up. Do your best to limit the time that you are soothing them so they don't become too dependent on you to get back to sleep.

A bedtime that is too early or too late is another cause of nightly wakings. It's easy to tell when your baby's bedtime is too early because they will wake up in the mood to play. It's important to not play with your baby when they wake up in the middle of the night as they will think it's time to get up. Instead, try to rock them or caress their cheek to ease them back to sleep.

If sleep training is inconsistent, your baby is more likely to wake up during the night. They need a routine that follows the same timings every day for their body to get used to sleeping through the night. If the routine is inconsistent, your baby will learn bad sleeping habits and they will continue to wake up during the night.

The best way to reduce night wakings is to develop a calm and consistent bedtime routine that works for you and your family. Make sure you have identified the strategies that work to help get your baby to sleep during the night, such as turning on white noise or closing the blinds.

When it comes to your baby, you also need to follow your instincts. You need to be comfortable with the strategies you use to get your baby back to sleep. If you're uncomfortable with a certain strategy, chances are they are too.

Where should your baby sleep?

Truthfully, no one can tell you where the best place for your baby to sleep is. You can decide to co-sleep or you can place them in their own room. While it is always best for your baby to be in their own crib and room when they are sleep training, this is not always possible. Sometimes you have space issues and do not have enough room in another bedroom for your baby, so they remain in yours until you can find a bigger place. Other times it is better to keep your baby in your bedroom for other reasons, especially if your baby tends to get sick often or your older children could disrupt the baby's sleep. You can decide to place a crib or bassinet into your room. This allows your baby to be next to you but gives them their own space. It is important to remember that just because your baby is in your room, does not mean they need to sleep in your bed.

You might also feel that co-sleeping with your baby in your bed is simply your parenting style. You do not want to place your baby in their own bed or even their own room until they tell you that they are ready, which might be around two years old.

If you do decide to co-sleep with your baby, you might look into products such as DockATot. This product helps separate your baby by placing them in a spot on your bed that will keep them from any dangers, such as falling into cracks between the bed and wall or heavy blankets getting on top of them. However, you should be aware that DockATot is not approved for safe sleeping because your baby can suffocate if they get too close to the padding during the night.

If you want the safest option for co-sleeping, you want to look at attaching a little crib right next to your bed. This gives you easy reach when you need to dream feed or your baby wakes up. It also gives them the sensation of being in their own bed, yet they are still co-sleeping.

Even though co-sleeping is a favorite for most parents, at least for a certain period of time, there is nothing safer than letting your baby sleep in their own crib. Even if the crib is in your room, it allows you to control their sleeping space the best and can eliminate as many risks as possible.

To give you a run down, here are the pros and cons of cribs:

Pros	Cons
As long as you have a crib that is recently made, it will meet all the safe sleeping standards for babies.	When your baby cries, you need to get out of bed to take care of them.
You can sleep without worrying about covers and pillows covering up your baby or them falling between any cracks.	You need to get up to check on your baby throughout the night.
Your baby will learn to sleep independently starting at a young age.	Your baby can try to climb out of the crib when they are older, which can cause them to harm themselves.

No matter what you decide, the most important factor that should influence your decision is your baby's safety. Over 3,500 babies die every year due to sleep-related deaths, such as SIDS, suffocating, and strangulation (Should Baby Sleep in a Crib or Co-Sleep with Mom and Dad,

2019). These statistics are not here to scare you, but to make you aware that it can happen.

To help you make your baby's sleeping space the safest for them, here are a few tips from the American Academy of Pediatrics:

- Place your baby's crib into your room as this is known to reduce SIDS by 50%.

- Lay your baby on their back when they sleep.

- Do not place blankets, pillows, and stuffed animals around your baby's sleeping surface. Their sleeping area needs to be firm and clear of anything that can cover their face or strangle them.

- Do not drink or smoke when you are caring for your baby. Do not allow other people to smoke around your baby.

- Do not share a sleeping surface with your baby.

- You can use pacifiers.

Chapter 10: Baby First Year and Beyond

Your baby's first year is full of milestones. There is nothing like watching your newborn develop into a toddler. You will have many milestones throughout your baby's day, some of which you will not even be aware of. For example, you will never truly know how much your baby takes in and learns throughout their day. You will notice when they start to grab on to their bottle while feeding or when they start to roll over. You will notice when they sit up by themselves and start to crawl. You will hear their coos develop into words, but you will not hear their thoughts. You will not know everything they are taking in mentally. When they become older, you will not fully be aware of how much their brain works every day—which is harder than ours because their brain is still developing.

Not every moment of parenthood will be its greatest, but you can take every moment as you wish. In a perfect world, every day will be full of perfectly huggable moments. But, we do not live in a perfect world and you will need to take the stressful and chaotic moments along with the huggable moments. This is okay as it is a part of parenthood and one factor you need to prepare yourself for. After all, every moment is what you make of it. There are parents who take the chaotic moments and use them as learning experiences. There are parents who take every moment and do their best to remain calm and smile through it because they realize one day these moments will be gone as well. Your child grows quickly, trust me. Before you know it, they will be ready for their first day of school. You will enroll them in the youth group at your local church. They will start going out with friends during Halloween. And soon, you will have a senior on your hands, and you are preparing their high school graduation and sending them off to college.

But, for now, it is time to focus on their first year and learn to enjoy every moment as much as possible.

Keys to Start Your Schedule

When it comes to your baby, their needs are not too difficult to understand, which is one reason you will have people telling you that the first year is the easiest during your parenting journey. There will be moments throughout your child's life where you do wish they were a baby again—at least I have had these moments. However, when you are in your child's first year, especially if this is your first baby, it seems like some of the hardest moments of your life. No matter how you feel, it is important to note that your baby loves you and they are dependent on you. They trust that you will feed them, clothe them, love them, and take care of them. They need the basics at this point and even when you feel the most overwhelmed, you are the best person for your child and you are an excellent mother.

The biggest struggle for most parents is knowing what your baby needs and when and how to balance your baby's needs and the needs of your other family members. On top of this, you still need time with your friends, alone time, and to attend to your other needs. There are times that you will feel that this balance is nearly impossible, but you will do your best and make it through every moment.

One of the reasons parents start a routine with their baby is because it does make life easier, especially during the first year. This not only helps you when it comes to finding a balance within your life, but you will know what your baby needs because they will learn what comes next. For example, they will know it is time to burp after they eat and then you will change their diaper. If you take a few minutes longer to change their diaper, they will start to inform you that they are waiting, and it is time to change their diaper. Tanya Remer Altmann states that babies like to know what is going to happen next because it helps them feel more secure. She also states schedules help you because when your baby is "not sleep-deprived or hungry, it makes for a much happier baby. By meeting your baby's basic needs, you put her in the best frame of mind – and body – to learn about and explore her new world" (Montgomery, 2019).

Starting a schedule with your baby will also help you continue the routine as they grow. You will find yourself changing parts of the routine, such as changing bedtime and the number of naps they take.

Another benefit of starting a routine with your baby is it will give them an easier transition when they are left with a babysitter or caregiver. For example, they will feel more comfortable at daycare because they know this is part of their routine. They will also establish a routine at daycare and begin to learn when you will pick them up. Leaving your baby with a babysitter can be a scary time for them because they do not always know the person. However, by talking to your babysitting about their routine and making sure they are on the same page, the transition will go a little more smoothly. Your baby might still cry when you leave, but they will quickly turn their attention to the next task with their babysitter.

When should you start your baby on a schedule?

Experts are quick to weigh in on when you should start your baby on a schedule. As you read through everything the experts say, you might become overwhelmed and wonder what the right step to take is. Similar to starting your baby on sleep training, you need to do what feels right. If you are trying to follow a schedule, but it is making you feel a little uneasy your baby will start to notice this feeling and think that something is wrong. This will cause them to feel uneasy and become upset.

Pediatrician Harvey Karp states that everyone is a creature of habit, even babies. They are their happiest when they are on a routine because they know what is coming next. Their routine becomes their habit and they are comfortable.

It is important for you to note that your baby will have a natural pattern to their day. If you want to work with your baby on developing the best routine, then you want to observe their daily structure. You can track the times they seem most alert and ready to interact and play, when they want to eat, sleep, and even when they need a diaper change. For example, a friend of mine once told me, "I know when it is almost time to leave the house because I will need to change my baby's messy diaper." It is true, babies will have a pooping schedule just like they have a feeding schedule. I had someone tell me once that they started to set their alarm for 1:00 a.m. because they knew their baby needed a diaper change.

As a busy mama, you probably wonder what the best way to track your baby's schedule is, as using a notepad might not work for you. Fortunately, there are a lot of apps that you can download on your smartphone, iPad, or find online using your computer. Some of these apps are Bundle Baby, Trixie Tracker, and Feed Baby.

To help you establish a routine with your little one, there are three main routine groups for you to focus on:

1. **Baby-led schedules.** This type of schedule does not have a strict definition or a lot of guidelines because you basically follow your baby when it comes to setting their routine. You will track what they need and when and start to find patterns. From this, you can get ahead and know that in 15 minutes your baby will want to eat. You will know that about an hour after they burp, they will need a diaper change. While this might make your days feel a little unpredictable in the first couple of weeks, once you start to find patterns, you will develop a strong routine with your baby. However, this type of scheduling can be tricky because your baby might have a different routine

depending on the day. For instance, they might need a diaper change anytime between 3:00 p.m. and 4:30 p.m. They might get hungry anytime between 11:30 a.m. and 1:00 p.m. These are factors that you will need to deal with the best you can. For instance, you have a varied time your baby will be hungry, so you can focus on setting a target time for feeding. You might track your baby's routine for a few weeks and decide they ate most of the time around 12:15 p.m. and establish this as your target time.

2. **Parent-led schedules.** This type of schedule is very strict as it is up to you to set times for everything. For example, you will not only set a naptime, but you will also set a certain amount of time for how long your baby naps. You might follow your baby's patterns through observation, but once you put everything in place, your schedule is set and you remain consistent, down to the minute. You might set a

timer that will tell you that it is time to get your baby up from their nap. Of course, there are some factors, such as diaper changes, that you cannot control. You also might let them sleep longer when they are sick or simply overtired. Gina Ford is an advocate for this type of schedule and commonly writes about it.

3. **Combination schedule.** I know many parents who tend to follow a combination of parent-led and baby-led schedules. While they set some of the timeframes and when their baby lays down for a nap, they do not follow it down to the minute. They are consistent, but also take it day by day. For example, if their baby is teething, they might allow them to sleep a little longer throughout the day as this lets their baby catch up on sleep— sometimes them as well. Sometimes parents will push back the nap because their baby is not tired enough to sleep yet. This doesn't mean that they will skip the

nap or wait a half an hour. Chances are your baby will get tired enough within a few minutes and then they will be ready for their nap.

You should also note that it is fine to lay your baby down for a few minutes if they are overtired and seem to need a little cat nap. It is important to make sure your baby can make it to their bedtime, which is the purpose of a cat nap. Most cat naps are about 20 to 45 minutes long, so they are usually a shorter length of time than their regular naps.

No matter when you decide to start the routine, the best option for you is to trust your instincts and listen to your baby. You will soon understand what they are trying to tell you and be able to know when they are hungry and when they are tired.

Newborn Days

When you have a newborn you often wonder if you will ever get a full night's sleep again. The answer to this question is yes! You will get a full night's sleep. In fact, sooner than you think if you start sleep training your baby. However, with a newborn, there are a few months to wait before you start sleep training. This does not mean that you cannot get a start on the routine as every baby, from the time they are born, should have a daily schedule that is consistently followed.

Zero to Six Weeks Newborn: Sleep Schedule

The sleep schedule for your newborn is rather erratic and does not seem to have a set pattern. This is typical for newborns as they will mainly sleep throughout the 24-hour period. They can easily sleep 16 hours a day but will normally not go over that amount of time. Newborns will often be awake when they are eating, and you can find their eyes looking all around their environment as they are trying to take in everything they can.

Brittney Stefanic from Brittney Stefanic Sleep Consulting states that newborns are unable to stay awake for over 40 minutes. This means that your newborn is pretty much awake for their feeding, getting cleaned up, and changing. Once they get to the point where you are ready to change their outfit, they are pretty much ready for another nap.

A typical day for your sleepy newborn looks a bit like this:

- The day for your newborn should start between 6:00 to 6:30 a.m.

- Your newborn should sleep a total of 14 to 16 hours in a 24-hour period.

- Your newborn should take about three to four naps per day. Each nap is usually between 30 minutes to 3 hours in length.

- Your newborn will be awake between 45 minutes to two hours between each sleep.

- The longest amount of time they will sleep at once is between three to six hours.

- Your newborn's bedtime should be between 8:00 to 10:00 p.m.

Parents and experts agree that the biggest challenge when it comes to the 0-6 week mark is you feel that you are in a sleep and poop cycle. You will wonder if your baby will ever become a bit more active. Trust me, they will. Before you know it, your baby will start to coo and demand your attention when they want it. Brittney Stefanic states to help your baby during this time with the day and night confusion, "One of the best ways to clear up the day/night confusion...is to expose baby to natural light during the daytime and keep them in a dark room during the night to allow their circadian rhythm and hormone levels to start to adjust to life outside the womb" (Baby Sleep Simplified: Newborn Sleep Schedules + Patterns, n.d.)

Do not worry about having a structured sleep schedule at this age because your newborn still has their days and nights confused. The fact is, they need to sleep when they need it and they need to eat when they are hungry.

Two to Three Months: Baby Sleep Schedule

During this period, your baby's sleep pattern will start to become noticeable. You might notice that they tend to be up for half an hour between their sleep sessions during the night and then about an hour and a half during the day. You are also starting to notice your baby's signs that tell you they are sleepy.

Brittney Stefanic states the most important factor to remember when your baby is between their sleep sessions is a full feeding. They are typically only up for a little over an hour, which means you do not want to wait too long to feed your baby.

A typical day for your two to three-month-old will look like this:

- You should start the day around 6:00 to 6:30 a.m.

- The total hours of sleep your baby should get in a 24-hr period is 14 to 16 hours.

- Your baby should take three to four naps every day. Each nap should be about 30 minutes to three hours long.

- The time awake between sleep for your baby is about 45 minutes to two hours.

- The longest amount of time your baby will sleep in one stretch during the night is three to six hours.

- Your baby's bedtime should be between 8:00 to 10:00 p.m.

The biggest challenge you will face during this time is the amount of sleep you have been running on. You are tired, in fact, you are exhausted. You are coming off of the six week stretch of feeding your baby every few hours and you are praying that they will start to sleep for a longer period of time soon. Fortunately, you are over the hump and your baby will start to sleep for longer stretches.

One reason your baby will start to sleep a bit longer, and continue to increase this amount of time, is because their stomach is growing. They will stay full for a longer time frame, allowing you a longer break between feedings.

Another reason is that your baby is getting in a routine, which means you should start to take notes. You want to note what makes your baby soothe themselves to sleep. For example, does your baby like to be swaddled or do they enjoy having a little white noise playing in the background? Note all the times they eat, when they sleep, and for how long. When does your baby want to be a little more active and playful? You should note anything you feel can help you set a daily routine for your little one.

Four to Six Months: Baby Sleep Schedule

Between four to six months is when your baby's sleep schedule will start to change. This happens because they are starting to sleep longer duration and because you will start sleep training. The schedule for your four to six-month-old baby should hold these factors:

- Your baby's day should start between 7:00 to 8:00 a.m.

- In a 24-hour period, your baby should sleep a total of 12 to 15 hours.

- Your baby should not take more than three naps, with each nap between one to three hours long.

- The time awake between their periods of sleep should be between 1 ½ to 2 ½ hours long.

- The longest amount of time they will sleep in one setting is between four to eight hours. This length of time will become longer once they are sleep trained.

- You should put your baby to bed between 8:30 to 9:30 p.m.

The number of naps your baby takes during this time will depend on your baby. You might deal with a baby that simply does not want to take naps or you might have one that enjoys their two naps during the day. If you have a baby who is a bit tougher when it comes to their naps, here are a few tips to help you:

- Set your baby in their sleeping space once they start to tell you that they are tired. Remember, you want them to be drowsy, but not asleep.

- Does your baby have time to calm themselves from any chaos of the day or playing? A calm baby will be able to fall asleep easier.

- Look around at your baby's environment. Is there anything that might be scaring them or making them stay awake because they are interested in the object. For example, many parents like to place lights in their baby's room that shows stars or animals. Sometimes the colors change with these objects and this can keep your baby interested in the pattern. Even though it repeats, they will fight sleep because this is their favorite show to watch.

The biggest challenge you will face with your baby is their transitions. These are hard on your precious bundle of joy because babies do not like change. It makes them worry about what will happen next and they do not feel as secure as they once did. While they know that everything will be okay because you are there, they still worry. The biggest key to working with your baby through their transitions is to be patient and understand that they are dealing with a big change in their life. Their transition might seem small to you, but to them, it is the most important factor happening in their life right now.

Feeding has come down a little bit by this stage. While they will eat about five to six times throughout the day, they might only need one nighttime feeding. Through your sleep training and dream feeding, you might be able to eliminate this nighttime feeding within a week or so.

Six to 10 Months: Baby Sleep Schedule

Your baby is unique. Your baby is different from all the other babies in the world and you need to hold this uniqueness with pride. Their personality is starting to show and with this comes the way they handle their sleep training and schedule. While your baby might have a bit of a different schedule, the basics are as follows:

- Your baby's day should begin at about 7:00 in the morning.

- Your baby should sleep about 11 to 15 hours in a 24-hour period.

- Your baby should have two or three naps, each at a length of one to three hours.

- Your baby should be awake two to three hours between each of their periods of sleep.

- The longest stretch of sleep your baby will have during the night is five to 10 hours.

- You should put your baby to bed between 8:30 to 9:30 p.m.

Unless you have already mastered the art of sleep training, your biggest challenge is getting your baby to sleep through the night. Because most parents start to sleep train at the beginning of this stage, it does not seem like a challenge for long. However, you need to remember that your little one will wake up a couple of times throughout the night and this is normal. They might self-soothe themselves to sleep or they might need you to come in and help them.

This is around the time you will start adding solid foods to your baby's diet. This can mess with their diaper changing schedule if they have one. It can also cause them to feel a little fussier from time to time as their body starts to adjust to the solid foods. Usually, the first step is adding rice to their formula. Another way people start introducing their baby to solid foods is baby food, such as Gerber. One nice factor about bringing in solid foods is your baby will start sleeping a little longer during the night, especially if you give them rice milk before they fall asleep. At the same time, they will still drink breast milk or formula about five times throughout the 24-hour period.

10 to 12 Months: Baby Sleep Schedule

Starting about the 10-month mark is when you will start to notice your baby is following your sleep schedule a little more closely. They are awake more during the day, though still on at least one nap, if not two, and sleeping for a longer period at night. If you have sleep trained, your baby could easily be sleeping through the night with brief wake times where they are typically able to soothe themselves back to sleep. However, this is also the time of teething, which can definitely disrupt their sleep for your baby and you.

The biggest challenge you will have at this age is the possibility of setbacks. Your baby can fall into sleep regression and separation anxiety. For example, you leave your baby in their crib like normal. You have successfully sleep trained them, so you expect that they will fall asleep without a problem, especially because they are drowsy. You notice them watching you as you walk out of their bedroom, but you do not think much of this until you shut the door and they immediately start crying. This is not a soft whimper like they usually do or a little cry, it is almost their cry that they are scared and need you now. Of course, you head back in to calm your little one and notice that they quickly calm down. You lay them back down again, shut the door, and it repeats. If this happens, your baby might have hit the separation anxiety stage and they believe that once you leave their room and shut the door, you are gone. Because they can no longer see you, you are no longer there. Even if you are in the next room, they believe that you are gone.

This is a frustrating time for you, but it is normal for your baby. Whether you are experiencing separation anxiety or a sleep setback, Brittney Stefanic gives the following advice:

> "Responding with consistency and holding your baby to their personal best is a great way to overcome sleep setbacks as quickly as possible. It is important to minimize the confusion that our children experience by staying consistent in the messages we send them, in sleep and beyond!" (Baby Sleep Simplified: Newborn Sleep Schedules + Patterns, n.d.).

A typical day for this age looks as follows:

- Your baby's day should start between 6:00 to 7:30 a.m.

- In a 24-hour period, your baby will sleep a total of 11 to 14 hours.

- Your baby might be down to one longer two-hour nap after lunch, or they might take two one hour naps during the day. Either way, naps are normally between one to two hours in length.

- Your baby will start to stay away between 2 ½ to 3 ½ hours between their sleep sessions. They can stay up a little longer.

- Your baby's longest stretch of sleep at night should be between seven to 12 hours.

- Your baby's bedtime should be between 8:00 and 9:00 p.m.

When it comes to feeding, your baby should only bottle feed about three to four times every day.

You will start to alternate between the bottle and solid foods. About 10 months old, you might start to notice your baby becoming hungrier. This is because your baby is also become a bit more active, such as crawling around wherever they can go or even starting to pull themselves up on furniture and walk along with the furniture. You might also help them walk around your home or set them in a walk so they can carry on as they wish. Their increase in activity means they will need more calories. Follow your baby's need to eat and feed them when they are hungry. They will help you develop a new feeding schedule.

12 to 18 Months: Schedule and Transitions

Between the ages of 12 to 18 months, your baby will amaze you with everything they are picking up. They are starting to talk, walk, and reaching so many other milestones that it is hard to keep up with them. Sometimes you will take this rather literally as while they have little legs, they can definitely run once they have learned.

This is another major transition time for your baby because they continue to grow and learn so much. However, this also means that they can struggle when it comes to sleep. To make sure your growing baby turning toddler is transitioning well, you want to make sure that they are continuing to get the sleep they need. This might mean that you will change their sleeping routine a bit. For instance, because they are attached to you and still struggling with separation anxiety, they will want to hold your hand or have you lay with them until they fall asleep. While this is sometimes a challenge for you as you have work you want to get done after they go to bed or want to take your time to be alone and relax (this is more important than housework), you need to tend to your child. Fortunately, you will help your baby through their sleep regressions and transitions the best way you can simply by being there for them.

If your baby did not go through a sleep regression between 10 and 12 months, they will most likely hit one at this stage. This is also the stage where they will change from two naps, if they are still on two naps, to one nap.

12 to 18 months of sleep schedule

Your baby's sleep schedule will depend on whether they have one or two naps during the day. Before we break down the schedule depending on the number of naps, let's take a look at the basics of the sleep schedule.

- The average time your baby will be awake in between their sleep sessions is four to six hours.

- The total number of hours they will nap during the day is two to three. It does not matter if your baby takes one nap or two, you want to make sure they sleep a total of two to three hours.

- They should sleep a total of 11 to 14 hours a day. The amount of sleep your baby will need will depend on them. You might also note that they sleep closer to 14 hours in a 24 hour period when they are 12 and 13 months, but when they start to reach 14 to 15 months, they start decreasing how much they sleep and do not need a second nap.

If your baby takes one nap during the day, their daily schedule will look similar to this:

- Your baby should start their day at about 7 to 7:30 a.m. They should stay awake for about 4 ½ to 5 hours.

- Your baby should go down for a nap at about 12:00 p.m. They should nap for about two to three hours.

- Make sure to get your baby up about 2:00 p.m. or a little later. You might go by how tired they were, how well or poorly they slept the night before, or what their typical nap schedule is. They should stay awake for about five hours.

- You should put your baby to bed between 7:30 to 8:00 p.m. This will allow them to sleep about 11 or so hours, whether they wake up or not.

Following this schedule, even if your times are a little different, will allow your baby to get the amount of sleep they need. For example, if you need to get your baby up for daycare at 6:30 a.m., you will want to put them to bed between 6:30 and 7:00 p.m.

If your baby takes two naps during the day, their daily schedule will look similar to this:

- You should wake your baby up about 6:00 a.m., providing they are not already up and ready to eat and play. They should be up for about three hours.

- Your baby should lay down for their first nap at about 9:00 a.m. They should sleep for around 45 minutes.

- You should wake your baby up by 9:45 a.m. and allow them to be up for 3 to 3 ½ hours.

- Your baby should lay down for their second nap at 1:00 p.m. They should sleep for about one hour and 45 minutes.

- Make sure your baby is up by 3:45 p.m. and allow them to be up for 4 to 4 ½ hours.

- Your baby should go to bed around 8:00 p.m. They should sleep about 10 hours or more with or without waking up during the night.

This schedule will give your baby a total sleep time of 11 to 14 hours during a 24 hour period.

12 to 18 months of feeding schedule

The feeding schedule for your 12 to 18 months old baby will also change. For instance, you might decrease or stop breastfeeding altogether because they are getting the nutrients they need from other foods. Therefore, your nutrients are not necessary anymore. You can follow the breastfeeding schedule of what is best for your family or you can choose to continue breastfeeding to provide your baby with more nutrients and bonding time. While there is debate on how long you should breastfeed your baby, there are mothers who breastfeed until their children are two or three and some who will stop a few months after their baby is born. Sometimes your baby will tell you when they are ready to be done with breast milk.

Around one year old is when your baby will start switching to cow's milk, providing you drink this type of milk. When you make the switch, it is best to discuss it with your baby's pediatrician as some babies will not drink straight cow's milk as they are not used to it (other babies will love it and not get enough!) To help ease your baby into drinking cow's milk, you want to purchase whole milk and mix it in with your baby's formula. You can start by mixing a bottle of ¾ formula and ¼ whole milk. Once your baby enjoys that, go half and half and then add more whole milk than formula. Soon, your baby will be strictly on whole milk. If you do not drink cow's milk because you follow a vegan diet, talk to your baby's doctor to see what the best substitute is for them.

18 Months to 3 Years: Schedule and Transitions

Though you will always consider your baby a baby, they are technically now a toddler and seem to be getting into *everything*. Their curiosity is more than you can handle from time to time, but they are still the most adorable child you have ever seen in your life and watching them grow is one of life's greatest treasures. One of my favorite parts about this age is you can start to notice when they are observing and learning. You will catch on to their facial expressions as they stop to smell the flowers. They are a little slow to walk and move around at this age, for the most part anyway, because their minds are constantly going as they are taking everything that is new to them. Always remember, even when you are in a rush, to allow your child to stop and learn. While we have seen a bee inside a flower several times, this is the first time for them and it is an exciting moment.

Your child's schedule will continue to change as they grow. You will also learn that you will change their bedtime routine up a little as they become more interactive. For example, one of my friends sang a lullaby to her baby until about the age of two. During this time, their toddler began to ask them to read a story. Therefore, my friend decided to read instead of sing and she continues to read to her toddler every night.

From the age of 18 months until three years old, the amount of sleep your toddler needs will change. A one-year-old, which includes an 18-month-old, needs 11 to 14 hours of sleep. A two-year-old needs 12 to 12 ½ hours every 24-hours. A three-year-old might still sleep about the same amount of time, but they will also start to drop their nap. However, some toddlers will continue to nap, at least for an hour every day, until the age of four.

Unless your toddler has a medical problem, wakes up from a dream, is sick, or starts teething again (they do start getting their molars between 18 months and 2 years old), they should sleep well throughout the night. Part of this is your sleep training while another part is because of their age.

Just because your toddler is most likely to sleep through the night does not mean they will not ever wake up during the night. Other than the reasons above, there are several reasons your toddler might find themselves awake. For example, you might have a new addition to the family and the baby wakes up your toddler. While you try to stop this, it is bound to happen and it is best you accept it and help your toddler understand the difference between a baby and themselves. If your toddler gets out of bed and wants to help you with the baby, you can allow this. Giving them a job to do is more likely to calm their minds and prepare them to fall back asleep quickly when they lay down. Your toddler might also wake up because it happens. It happens to adults and it will happen to toddlers too.

Because every toddler is different, it is hard to give you one schedule that your toddler should follow. Therefore, there are three different schedules below. You want to use one of these schedules as a guideline for your toddler. For example, you might put your toddler to bed half an hour earlier because they need to get up earlier. If this happens, it means that your time will always be a half of an hour ahead.

Toddler schedule number one: two naps

Your 18-month-old can easily be on the two nap schedule. By the time your child turns two, they should go down to one nap during the day. Until this point, here is a guideline for their sleep and feeding schedule.

- You will want to wake your child up by 7:00 a.m.

- Feed your child right away as they will be hungry from a full night's sleep. Breakfast should be no later than 7:30 a.m.

- Your toddler is growing, and they will get hungry making 9:30 a.m. a great time to give your child a light snack. You do not need to give them a snack if they are not hungry. For instance, if they are not in a growth spurt, they might not care for a snack. Yet, they might want a snack every day because they feel it is part of their routine.

- Lay your child down for their morning nap at 10:00 a.m. They should sleep for no more than one hour.

- Feed your child lunch between 11:30 a.m. and 12:00 p.m.

- Lay your toddler down for their afternoon nap at 2:00 p.m. Again, they should not sleep longer than one hour.

- Around 3:30 p.m. is a great time to give your little one an afternoon snack as they will be hungry by this time.

- You should feed your child supper around 5:30 p.m. This will allow them to have a little quiet playtime before the bedtime routine begins.

- Start your toddler's bedtime routine around 6:30 p.m.

- Your toddler should go to bed at about 7:00 p.m.

Toddler schedule number two: one nap

This schedule is similar to the first schedule, but it only has one nap during the day.

- Your toddler should get up by 7:00 a.m.

- You want to feed your toddler breakfast by 7:30 a.m.

- If your toddler needs a light snack, a great time to feed them is 9:00 a.m.

- Your baby should eat lunch at 11:00 a.m.

- Lay your little one down or a nap by 12:00 p.m. They should sleep for at least one hour. Because they only have one nap during the day, they might sleep closer to two hours, but should not go beyond that as it will be harder for them to fall asleep at night.

- Feed your toddler an afternoon snack about 3:30 p.m.

- Have dinner ready for your child at 5:30 p.m.

- Let your toddler quietly play until you begin their bedtime routine at 6:30 p.m.

- Shut off the lights and make sure your toddler knows it is time to go to bed at 7:00 p.m.

Toddler schedule number three: no nap

Your toddler will eventually stop taking naps altogether. This might come on gradually when you begin to notice that it is harder for your little one to fall asleep at night or because your child's pediatrician believes it is time to cut out naps completely so your child sleeps better at night. It is always best to follow your child's direction when it comes to taking away their nap. If you take it away too soon, your baby won't get the amount of sleep they need in a 24-hour period and this can cause them to become irritable, moody, and lead to other consequences.

- Wake up time for your toddler should be at 7:00 a.m.

- Similar to the other schedules, you want to feed your little one by 7:30 a.m.

- The best time to feed your child a light snack, if they are hungry, is at 9:30 a.m.

- Have lunchtime with your child at 12:00 p.m.

- Instead of giving them a nap at 1:00 p.m. you should instead have quiet or rest time. This is not a time for them to fall asleep, though they might from time to time. It allows them to transition better from a nap to no naps. It can also give you a much-needed break after a busy morning. This time should not last longer than an hour.

- The best time for an afternoon snack is 3:30 p.m.

- Sit down to have dinner with your little one at 5:30 p.m.

- You should start their bedtime routine at 6:30 p.m.

- Make sure your toddler knows that it is time for them to go to bed at 7:00 p.m.

Chapter 11: The Secret Sauce and Fine Tuning

So, what is the secret sauce when it comes to sleep training your baby? From one mom to another who has used her experience and research to help you, it is consistency. There is no escaping this fact. The more consistent you are with your methods, no matter what method you choose, the easier your baby will catch on to sleep training, self-soothing, and before you know it everyone will sleep well throughout the night.

Along with consistency, there are other ingredients that go into the secret sauce:

- You can wake a sleeping baby. It is okay to do this, especially when they are sleeping too long during their naptime. You want them to stay on their schedule.

- Set a bedtime that will allow your baby to get enough sleep during the night. This means you need to consider the time you need to wake them up if you have to bring them to daycare.

- Establish a naptime routine that is different from a bedtime routine, so your baby learns it is time to nap and not bedtime.

- Be comfortable with your sleep training method and follow your instincts. Let your baby guide you if this is what you prefer.

"But I Have Tried Everything!" (Training Tools for the Exhausted Parent)

I have been there and I know many other parents who have felt the same way—you have tried everything and absolutely nothing has worked.

I understand exactly what you are saying. Take a deep breath and know that I am here to help.

You have tried several methods and your child is still waking up. You are consistent, patient, and still, nothing works. What else can you do?

- **Bedtime fading** means you will move your child's bedtime to a later time. For example, you notice that your baby cries for about an hour before they fall asleep. Therefore, you decide to push bedtime back 45 minutes. If this still does not work, you push it back another 15 minutes to make up for that whole hour. When your child starts to fall asleep within 10 to 15 minutes, you can start moving the bedtime up to an early time by 10 to 15 minutes.

- **Avoid the late sleep.** Babies can be a bit sneaky and try to get in a nap later in the day when you think they are playing quietly in the corner. If you notice your baby falling asleep, try to keep them up to their bedtime. If this is impossible, you can try to let them sleep for a few minutes, like a cat nap, but not much longer.

- **Camp out in your child's room.** When you camp out, you remain in your child's room until they fall asleep, but you slowly move closer to their doorway. You might move a little closer every night or decide to move closer as they are falling asleep. You need to watch them because if they start to get fussy, you want to move closer to them.

- **Bedtime chart.** If your child is older, it might work to have a bedtime chart where they can see their progress. Children love to play with stickers and allowing them to put a sticker on their chart in the morning can become a helpful tool.

10 Steps to Sleep Training Success

1. **Sleep is a priority.** Sleep training is a lifestyle, and this means that sleep becomes a priority. Always remember that your baby needs their sleep because their brain needs it. Without enough sleep, they will struggle to pay attention to what they need to learn.

2. **Get everyone on board.** Make an appointment with your baby's doctor, talk to anyone who cares for your baby and make sure that everyone understands the sleep training plan.

3. **Know the amount of sleep your baby needs.** You always want to watch your baby's age to make sure they are getting the right amount of sleep.

4. **Keep a journal.** You will not remember all the times your baby woke up, fell asleep, or when they ate, etc. So to help

you track their progress and note any patterns, you want to keep a journal. You can also use this to describe how well your baby handled sleep training.

5. **Ensure you have a routine.** You should create your routine before you start sleep training so you have everything in place for your start date.

6. **Have a start date.** Don't get up one morning and tell yourself that you will start sleep training your baby. The more planning you put into sleep training, the more successful it will be. This includes having a start date as this will allow you to prepare your baby's sleeping space, allow them to get used to anything you changed, and prepare yourself.

7. **Make sure you have the right environment for your baby.** You want to set the scene with a calming environment. This might include getting a

white noise machine or a few gentle music playlists.

8. **Put your baby down when they are awake.** You should place your baby in bed when they are still awake, yet sleepy. This will help them focus on their self-soothing techniques.

9. **Sit in a chair but move it away.** One method to follow when your baby is first learning the bedtime routine and training is to place a chair next to their crib. Sit there for a bit and then move the chair back a bit. Repeat this process until they are sleeping or you are at their doorway.

10. **Do not continue to use crutches.** Crutches are the soothing techniques that you use to put your baby to sleep. While you might still use them when your baby is sick or when they wake up and are inconsolable, you do not want to use them every night. This will make your baby

dependent on your soothing techniques and they will not learn to self-soothe.

Two main things you need to remember are that sleep training is a lifestyle and do not quit. I know you are stressed, and you feel that you have tried everything and *nothing* is working, but I will tell you something else—*you got this*. This is often easier to say than believe, but you will one day look back at your sleep training and realize all of the stress and realize that it is all worth it. You will be grateful that you did not quit, and you continued to work toward your goal.

The Reasons for Sleep Regression

There are times you thought you would never get a full night's sleep, but it finally happened. Your baby is successfully sleep trained. They are sleeping through the night, mostly self-soothing when they wake up and taking naps. They are happy and energetic. In fact, you believe they are more energetic now than they were before. However, so are you.

But then it happens. It is like your baby takes several steps back when it comes to sleeping. Your baby might be protesting their naps, or they might decide to wake up five times during the night and demand that you come and soothe them back to sleep. It is real. No matter what other people tell you, sleep regression is real.

First, you need to understand what the term means. Regression means that you go back to a previous state, such as your baby waking up five times throughout the night. When it comes to your baby and seemingly forgetting about self-soothing or their sleep training, it can be a blow to your system. But there is one factor that you need to keep in mind to understand why your child went into sleep regression mode—they are constantly growing, developing, and reaching milestones. This can have an effect on them that causes them to need you to soothe them for a period of time. They have not forgotten how to soothe themselves back to sleep, they simply need you during this time.

So what can you do to help your baby and yourself through sleep regression?

- Forget about the term regression.

- Start to call it "sleep transition" as this is what your baby is doing. They are transitioning to a new developmental stage.

- Realize this is normal. Every baby goes through sleep transitioning.

- Remember, this will pass. It is hard to remember this when you are on the sixth night of waking up four times with your baby at 10 months of age, but it is true. It will pass.

- Take a breather. If you need to ask someone to help you out, let them know. Just like when your baby was smaller, you can still reach out for help as you need to take care of yourself as well.

- Never forget—everything will fall into place for both you and your precious little one.

So now that we have talked a bit about sleep regression or transitioning, it is time to look at the causes.

1. **Physical developments.** It does not matter if your baby is learning or learned to sit, crawl, stand, or walk, they can all cause sleep regression. While there is little research done on it, some researchers believe the amount of time your baby is in sleep regression depends on when they learned the skill and if they learned early or later.

2. **Illness.** Your child getting sick, whether it is with a common cold or something more serious, has a lot to do with sleep regression. In reality, they simply need you to comfort them during this time.

3. **Traveling.** Babies are not like newborns. While newborns can sleep anywhere, babies struggle to sleep in a new place. If you are traveling, expect your baby to go into sleep regression mode.

4. **They are overtired.** It happens from time to time, your baby becomes overtired because of a long day or they simply haven't slept well lately.

5. **Stress or change within the family.** Most people think that their baby won't realize that there is a change within the family or when you are feeling stressed, but they can. They know when something is not the same and this causes them to feel insecure about their environment, bringing on a sleep regression episode.

6. **Switching to a big kid bed.** Your toddler will have trouble when it comes to making the transition between the crib to a new bed and this can cause them to struggle with sleep.

7. **Old habits are coming back.** It happens to the best of us. We are on a roll of developing new habits and soon, we find ourselves struggling and we start to bring back our old habits. The fact is, we usually do not realize that this is happening. Old habits can cause your baby to go into sleep regression mode.

Stages of sleep regression

Sleep regression can happen more than once and for many reasons. To help you better prepare for sleep regression episodes, here are the stages you need to keep in mind.

- **Four months.** At this stage, your baby might or might not be sleep trained. Whether they are or not, they will know self-soothing techniques and not often wake you up during the night because they woke up, until they start to go through their sleep regression. This comes on because they are going through so many developmental changes. Their sleeping patterns are changing, and they are more hungry because of a growth spurt.

- **Six months.** While nearly every baby will go through a four-month sleep regression, some will not go through a six-month regression. If your baby does, it is because they are learning how to crawl, stand next to furniture, or focusing on other physical developments.

- **Eight months.** In reality, this sleep regression can happen between eight to ten months, but most state it happens at about eight months. If your baby didn't crawl at six months, this could be the reason for their eighth-month regression. Other reasons are because they are learning more mentally than you realize. There is a lot going on within the mind of your child and this can make it hard for them to calm down and sleep.

Furthermore, separation anxiety starts around this age, which can also cause sleep regression.

- **One year.** At around one year of age, your baby will go through another sleep regression as they are learning how to walk. They might also start to nap less, which can also affect their regression.

- **18 months.** Your baby might not go through this stage, but if they do it is because of all their developmental changes. They are learning more skills, starting to talk, and their mind is becoming even more active. Furthermore, they are becoming more active physically, which can make them overtired.

While you may not completely stop all the sleep regression stages, there are a few tips that you can follow to help your baby and yourself through a sleep regression.

1. Continue to keep their sleep schedule. Yes, you might need to go in and soothe them more, but you want to continue to remain consistent when it comes to their daily schedule. The only time you will change their schedule is when they are dropping a nap.

2. Be patient and give your baby the comfort they need. Sleep regression is temporary, and they will work through it and continue on their sleep schedule in time.

3. Do not fall back into old habits. Do not allow your child to stay up later because they are highly active as this is also a sign of overstimulation. When this happens, it will be harder for your baby to fall asleep.

4. If you feel that you are at the end of your rope and you are in need of help, ask for help. You can use the same people who helped you when your baby was little or find different friends and family members. You might even contact a sleep

consultant. Of course, you can always find support through social media groups on Facebook.

Conclusion

I understand where you are now. You feel like you have tried everything, and you still cannot get your baby to sleep through the night. You are exhausted and you do not know where to turn. As a mother, I have the experience that can guide you in finding the best sleep training method for your baby, you, and your whole family. It does not matter if you are living with your partner or are a single parent, you have the skills and tools within this book to help your baby self-soothe themselves to sleep through your chosen sleep training method.

Throughout this book, we discussed several topics that pertain to sleep training. You know what sleep training is and you can prepare yourself for establishing a sleep training plan that will work for you and your baby. You know sleep training is a lifestyle and while it is hard, your baby will adjust as long as you are consistent and patient.

You now understand the harmful effects that sleep deprivation can have on your little one. It can affect them psychologically, emotionally, and physically. Sleep deprivation causes you to lose focus and patience. It can also lead to fatal consequences.

The contents of this book discussed how to sleep train with multiples, which inevitably brings a little more difficulty in the situation. But sleep training is still 100% doable with your twins as long as you continue to follow the golden rule of consistency along with the many other steps associated with sleep training.

You now know the seven types of cries and that there are many reasons why your child might be crying. There might be a reason that your child doesn't even understand or they simply just need a good cry. You know that while it seems daunting at first, you will learn your child's cries and communicate effectively with them.

You know that there is no reason to feel guilty or fear to try a sleep training technique. It is actually a helpful tool to help your child develop skills that they can continue to use throughout their life, such as self-discipline and soothing themselves.

There are no big secrets as to why sleep training fails. You know what to look out for and what you should avoid so you do not make some of the same mistakes parents before you have made.

You received information about two main methods when it comes to sleep training: the cry it out method and the no tears method. You should choose the method that best suits you and your baby. You need to be comfortable with the method as this will make your baby more comfortable as they learn the method.

There needs to be a difference between your child's naptime and their bedtime routine. You also want to make sure that you do not combine their feeding time with bedtime. All of these pieces of their day should remain separate as it will allow them to keep their schedules more easily.

You learned about the secret sauce that you need to make sure that your sleep training is successful. As long as you carry this secret sauce with you through the sleep training journey, your baby will get the sleep they need to begin to thrive even more throughout their day.

There is a lot of information that I want you to remember through this book, but the most important factor is that you need to know that you can do this. You are not alone and even though you feel like you have tried everything, you will become successful in your sleep training efforts. You are an amazing person and all of the tension you feel from a lack of sleep will pass. Believe in yourself because I believe in you. When you need to take a step back, do this. When you need to ask for help, do this. When you need to let out a good cry because you are so overwhelmed, this is okay too. But know that at the end of your day, you are doing your best and you should be proud.

Hello there Mommies,

Caring for your newborn brings great joy and excitement, but with it also comes sleep deprivation. It's a fact: Newborns simply can't sleep through the night, so neither can you.

The good news is that babies typically develop regular sleep patterns and can be put to sleep with help of a proper sleep-training As your baby's brain matures over these first few months, you'll probably see a sleep pattern start to emerge. Help your newborn establish a consistent sleep pattern by making routines for your baby's daily activities. In this way, you get back your sleep as well.

Track your baby's daily schedule for feeding, sleeping, crying and changing diapers. Once those patterns begin to form, you can help your baby settle into a daily routine and sleep pattern.

So, get you're your Your Baby Schedule Tracker " in PDF format by clicking the link below:

https://harleycarrparenting.com/you-and-your-baby-can-sleep-through-the-night/

+

QR Code

Print the document and start to record your Baby's daily Activities.

This Printable baby Schedule chart can help you identify patterns and figure out a routine that works for your baby and for the whole family.

Now, you can have your "Baby Schedule Tracker" in just one click away!

Let´s get started ...

Enjoy and Best Wishes to you Mommy!

Harley Carr

References

12 Steps to Sleep-Training Success. Retrieved 25 November 2019, from https://www.parents.com/baby/sleep/tips/ten-steps-to-sleep-training-success/

15 Ways Lack of Sleep Is Harmful To The Baby. (2016). Retrieved 17 November 2019, from https://www.babygaga.com/15-ways-lack-of-sleep-is-harmful-to-the-baby/

Alexander, L. (2019). Decoding Baby Crying (8 Types of Crying You Might Hear). Retrieved 7 December 2019, from https://momlovesbest.com/decoding-baby-crying

Baby Sleep Simplified: Newborn Sleep Schedules + Patterns. Retrieved 24 November 2019, from https://www.nestedbean.com/pages/baby-and-newborn-sleep-schedules-patterns

Begley, J. (2018). Top 10 Causes of Sleep Regressions. Retrieved 25 November 2019, from https://thebabysleepgeek.com/top-10-causes-of-sleep-regressions/

Bryant, A. (2019). The complete guide to nap training your baby. Retrieved 25 November 2019, from https://momlikeyoumeanit.com/nap-training/

Canapari, C. (2015). The Top Ten Sleep Training Mistakes (& How To Avoid Them). Retrieved 23 November 2019, from https://drcraigcanapari.com/sleep-training-mistakes-and-pitfalls/

Canapari, C. (2019). Sleep Training Tools and Methods for the Exhausted Parent. Retrieved 25 November 2019, from https://drcraigcanapari.com/at-long-last-sleep-training-tools-for-the-exhausted-parent/

Chitnis, R. (2019). How to Teach Baby to Self Sooth - Effective Tips & Benefits. Retrieved 25 November 2019, from https://parenting.firstcry.com/articles/effective-ways-to-train-your-baby-for-self-soothing/

Colic, reflux, flatulence, or allergy – Why is my baby crying?. (2018). Retrieved 23 November 2019, from https://www.lullame.com/blogs/blog/colic-reflux-flatulence-or-allergy-why-is-my-baby-crying

Decoding Baby Crying. (2019). Retrieved 22 November 2019, from https://www.whattoexpect.com/first-year/week-10/decoding-cries.aspx

DeJeu, E. (2014). 3 Steps to Help Your Partner Put Baby to Bed. Retrieved 6 December 2019, from https://www.babysleepsite.com/sleep-training/partner-put-baby-to-sleep-3-steps/

Ding, K. Baby sleep training: No tears methods. Retrieved 22 November 2019, from https://www.babycenter.com/0_baby-sleep-training-no-tears-methods_1497581.bc

Doucleff, M. (2019). Sleep Training Truths: What Science Can (And Can't) Tell Us About Crying It Out. Retrieved 25 November 2019, from https://www.npr.org/sections/health-shots/2019/07/15/730339536/sleep-training-truths-what-science-can-and-cant-tell-us-about-crying-it-out

Dubinsky, D. Baby sleep training: Cry it out methods. Retrieved 22 November 2019, from https://www.babycenter.com/0_baby-sleep-training-cry-it-out-methods_1497112.bc

Dubinsky, D. Baby sleep training: The basics. Retrieved 16 November 2019, from https://www.babycenter.com/0_baby-sleep-training-the-basics_1505715.bc

Elsevier. (2008, September 4). Loss Of Sleep, Even For A Single Night, Increases Inflammation In The Body. ScienceDaily. Retrieved December 1, 2019 from www.sciencedaily.com/releases/2008/09/080902075211.htm

Gorton, R. This expert wants you to know: Sleep regressions aren't real. Retrieved 25 November 2019, from https://www.mother.ly/child/what-a-sleep-expert-wants-tired-mamas-to-know-about-sleep-regressions

Harris, N. Baby Growth Charts: Birth to 36 Months. Retrieved 25 November 2019, from https://www.parents.com/baby/development/growth/baby-growth-charts-birth-to-36-months/

How to Deal With Crying Twin Babies. (2019). Retrieved 22 November 2019, from https://www.whattoexpect.com/first-year/baby-care/how-to-deal-with-crying-twin-babies/

How to Get Baby to Nap: Baby Nap Schedule During the 1st Year. Retrieved 24 November 2019, from https://www.nestedbean.com/blogs/zen-blog/how-to-get-baby-to-nap-baby-nap-schedule-during-the-1st-year?utm_source=page&utm_medium=intext&utm_campaign=newbornsleepschedules

Johnson, N. (2019). Toddler Sleep Schedules With Feedings. Retrieved 25 November 2019, from

https://www.babysleepsite.com/schedules/todd
ler-schedule/

Karp, H. How to Handle Your Baby's Night
Wakings. Retrieved 22 November 2019, from
https://www.happiestbaby.com/blogs/baby/bab
y-night-wakings-help

Karp, H. What Is Dream Feeding? And How Do I
Do It?. Retrieved 22 November 2019, from
https://happiestbaby.com.au/blogs/baby/what-
is-a-dream-feed-and-how-do-i-do-it

Martinelli, K. Finding a Sleep Training Method
That Works for Your Family. Retrieved 22
November 2019, from
https://childmind.org/article/choosing-a-sleep-
training-method-that-works-for-your-family/

Michi, R. (2017). Gentle Sleep Training- The
Role of Grandparents. Retrieved 14 November
2019, from
https://childrenssleepconsultant.com/2017/07/
24/gentle-sleep-training-the-role-of-
grandparents/

Michi, R. (2017). Gentle Sleep Training: The Role of Dads. Retrieved 14 November 2019, from https://childrenssleepconsultant.com/2017/07/13/gentle-sleep-training-the-role-of-dads/

Montgomery, N. (2019). The basics of baby schedules: Why, when, and how to start a routine. Retrieved 24 November 2019, from https://www.babycenter.com/0_the-basics-of-baby-schedules-why-when-and-how-to-start-a-rou_3658352.bc

Moye, J. (2018). Sleep Training's Simple, Effective Secret Weapon. Retrieved 6 December 2019, from https://www.fatherly.com/parenting/how-to-share-sleep-training-with-your-partner/

Newborn Baby Routine. Retrieved 23 November 2019, from https://www.tresillian.org.au/advice-tips/daily-activities/0-3-months/

Our Guide to Understanding Childhood Sleep Regression. (2017). Retrieved 25 November

2019, from https://www.tuck.com/sleep-regression/

Pennington, C. (2016). Caring for newborn twins or multiples. Retrieved 18 November 2019, from https://www.babycenter.com/0_caring-for-newborn-twins-or-multiples_3590.bc

Pyanov, M. (2017). Why The Feed-Play-Sleep Routine Doesn't Work For Breastfed Babies. Retrieved 25 November 2019, from https://www.bellybelly.com.au/baby/feed-play-sleep-routine-breastfed-babies/

Ruiz, R. (2016). Why new parents shouldn't feel so guilty about sleep training. Retrieved 25 November 2019, from https://mashable.com/2016/05/25/sleep-training-guilt-study/

Schiedel, B. (2019). Sleep and feeding schedule for your 12- to 18-month-old baby. Retrieved 25 November 2019, from https://www.todaysparent.com/baby/baby-sleep/12-to-18-month-old-schedule/

Setting Up Your Twins' Sleep Schedule. (2019). Retrieved 23 November 2019, from https://www.whattoexpect.com/first-year/baby-care/setting-up-your-twins-sleep-schedule.aspx

Should Baby Sleep in a Crib or Co-Sleep with Mom and Dad?. (2019). Retrieved 24 November 2019, from https://lambsivy.com/blogs/news/should-baby-sleep-in-a-crib-or-co-sleep-with-mom-and-dad

Smart Solutions for Baby's Nighttime Waking. Retrieved 22 November 2019, from https://www.sleep.org/articles/smart-solutions-for-babys-nighttime-waking/

The Best Routines for Twin Babies. (2018). Retrieved 21 November 2019, from https://www.whattoexpect.com/first-year/baby-care/the-best-routines-for-twin-babies.aspx

The Secret Sauce for Sleep Training Babies. (2019). Retrieved 25 November 2019, from https://fortworth.citymomsblog.com/2019/08/15/the-secret-sauce-for-sleep-training-babies/

Thompson, A. (2019). Make Sleep Training Easier By Involving Your Partner. Retrieved 14 November 2019, from https://adelethompsonsleepconsulting.com/make-sleep-training-easier-by-involving-your-partner/

Thompson, A. (2019). Make Sleep Training Easier By Involving Your Partner. Retrieved 21 November 2019, from https://adelethompsonsleepconsulting.com/make-sleep-training-easier-by-involving-your-partner/

Tweaking Your Toddler Twins' Routines. (2019). Retrieved 25 November 2019, from https://www.whattoexpect.com/first-year/baby-care/tweaking-your-toddler-twins-routines.aspx

Twins. (2019). Retrieved 22 November 2019, from https://www.basisonline.org.uk/twins/

What 'sleeping through the night' actually means. (2018). Retrieved 23 November 2019, from https://www.kidspot.com.au/baby/baby-care/baby-sleep-and-settling/what-sleeping-through-the-night-means/news-story/139696676cb12bb7459dba318decb95f

Your Twins' Bath Time. (2018). Retrieved 21 November 2019, from https://www.whattoexpect.com/first-year/baby-care/your-twins-bath-time.aspx

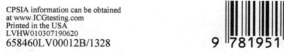